Praise

DON'T SWEAT THE S

"After almost two decades since the original release of *Don't Sweat the Small Stuff*, Richard Carlson's insights on the meaning of life continue to be timeless. The book teaches us to focus on the 'now' and find balance by living through contentment."

—Deepak Chopra

"Over a decade of positive psychology research seems to validate what we learned twenty years ago from *Don't Sweat the Small Stuff*. . . . These wonderful books help break down and simplify how to achieve that happiness."

—Shawn Achor, bestselling author of *The Happiness Advantage*

"Richard Carlson caused a revolution in all our thinking with his *Don't Sweat the Small Stuff* books. He was like a Zen master in disguise, taking almost an aw-shucks attitude toward shifting the culture."

—Marianne Williamson, *New York Times* bestselling author of *A Return to Love*

"Kristine Carlson is the real deal, a shining light guiding us away from the pitfalls of stress and despair, fear and anxiety, and illuminating the path to acceptance, happiness, and achieving your goals."

—Karen Salmansohn, bestselling author of *The Bounce Back Book*

"Reminds us with simple brilliance of what it takes to rise to our best and what we need to do to enjoy a life beautifully lived."

—Robin Sharma, bestselling author of *The Monk Who Sold His Ferrari*

"*Don't Sweat the Small Stuff* has the power to change our individual and collective lives. I am deeply grateful to Dr. Richard Carlson and his beloved wife Kristine for their wisdom and compassion in bringing transformational practices and perspectives to millions of readers."

—Shauna Shapiro, author of *The Art and Science of Mindfulness*

Don't Sweat *the* Small Stuff Every Day

Alexa!

Love you!

Kris

Don't Sweat *the* Small Stuff Every Day

365 SIMPLE WAYS
TO LIVE A LIFE YOU LOVE

RICHARD CARLSON
AND
KRISTINE CARLSON

Go
hachette
BOOKS
New York

Cover design by Amanda Kain

Material from this book was first published in:
Don't Sweat the Small Stuff in Love (2000)
Don't Sweat the Small Stuff at Work (1999)
Don't Sweat the Small Stuff About Money (2001)
Don't Sweat the Small Stuff... and It's All Small Stuff (1997)
Don't Sweat the Small Stuff with Your Family (1998)

Hachette Go, an imprint of Hachette Books
Hachette Book Group
1290 Avenue of the Americas
New York, NY 10104
HachetteGo.com
Facebook.com/HachetteGo
Instagram.com/HachetteGo

First Edition: December 2024

Published by Hachette Go, an imprint of Hachette Book Group, Inc. The Hachette Go name and logo is a trademark of the Hachette Book Group.

Print book interior design by Six Red Marbles

Library of Congress Control Number: 2024940967

ISBNs: 978-0-306-83526-1 (trade paperback); 978-0-306-83527-8 (ebook)

Printed in the United States of America

LSC-C

Printing 1, 2024

This book is dedicated to our grandchildren and their children with all our love.

Also available in the Don't Sweat the Small Stuff series

Don't Sweat the Small Stuff . . . and It's All Small Stuff
Don't Sweat the Small Stuff with Your Family
Don't Sweat the Small Stuff at Work
Don't Sweat the Small Stuff in Love
Don't Sweat the Small Stuff About Money
Don't Sweat the Small Stuff for Women
Don't Sweat the Small Stuff for Men

CONTENTS

INTRODUCTION

Dear Reader,

Don't Sweat the Small Stuff, for decades now, has been a generational series guiding millions of people toward a happier life. When we stop focusing on what doesn't matter—that's the small stuff—and spend the majority of our time and energy living into what we value most, that's when we begin to live our very best lives.

Seventeen years ago, just one week before my beloved husband, Dr. Richard Carlson, passed away suddenly from a pulmonary embolism, was the ten-year anniversary of the first *Don't Sweat the Small Stuff* book. Richard stood in the kitchen and said to me, "Kris, the beauty of what we've created with the Don't Sweat series is that every ten years there will be a whole new generation of people who will benefit from our books." This statement has proven to be true.

During times of overwhelm, and I'm sure you'll agree that we are collectively in one of those times right now, we search out ways to bring calm to our days. We often look to what we can change in our outer world to manage the unpredictability of life. But in order to cultivate a buoyant heart and mind, we have to be committed to practicing life in ways that will sustain our inner well-being. It is our inner experience that is most important to our happiness.

This new book, *Don't Sweat the Small Stuff Every Day*, will inspire you to focus on a teaching and a chapter each day that comes from one of the many books in the Don't Sweat the Small Stuff series. Each chapter will be like a string of warm lights to help guide you forward through any challenge and into a place within yourself that remains strong, resilient, and calm. These qualities, when nurtured, will sustain your happiness through even the most difficult of times.

Over the years, I have received hundreds of letters from readers who remind me that our books help soothe their internal fears and anxiety and assist in guiding them toward the kind of lasting contentment that comes from practicing life in happy ways every day. Their messages confirm that it is the choices we make for ourselves each day—the choice to be more present, to become responsive versus reactive, to align with a healthy outlook, to be grateful for what we have, and to put in place simple strategies for living better—that help us live our best lives today.

Now you have the best of the best chapters of the series right here. And whether you've read the Don't Sweat series or not, it doesn't matter. If you have read from the series previously, the teachings in each chapter will impact you today as much as they did when you read them before—and maybe even more, because you've grown wiser over time and can look forward to new insights and discoveries as you read with an open heart.

One of my favorite chapters and teachings is "Start the Day with Love, Live the Day with Love, End the Day with Love." You can use this book to get off to a peaceful and inspired start to your day. By reading a short chapter every day and applying that teaching, you will start to feel better in various aspects of your life.

I would also recommend making this book part of family or couple reading at night, maybe sparking a new tradition to give you more quality time together. It's wonderful to end your day focused on something that helps ignite that spark of gratitude and inspiration, allowing you to rest your head in peace on your pillow as you go to sleep at night.

Even though we are going through difficult times in the world right now, one thing has always remained true. Your inner world dictates the nature of your experience. I hope that this book helps you to keep perspective and to have an optimistic view of life on a daily basis. And I hope it feeds your heart and soul in ways that bring you deep inner peace and joy.

Happier days are here as you read on.

Treasure the gifts of life and love,
Kristine Carlson

1.

DON'T SWEAT THE SMALL STUFF

Often we allow ourselves to get all worked up about things that, upon closer examination, aren't really that big a deal. We focus on little problems and blow them way out of proportion. A stranger, for example, might cut in front of us in traffic. Rather than let it go and go on with our day, we convince ourselves that we are justified in our anger. We play out an imaginary confrontation in our mind.

Why not try to have compassion for the person and remember how painful it is to be in such an enormous hurry. This way, we can maintain our own sense of well-being and avoid taking other people's problems personally.

There are many similar, "small stuff" examples that occur every day in our lives. Whether we had to wait in line, listen to unfair criticism, or do the lion's share of the work, it pays enormous dividends if we learn not to worry about little things. So many people spend so much of their life energy "sweating the small stuff" that they completely lose touch with the magic and beauty of life. When you commit to working toward this goal, you will find that you have far more energy to be kinder and gentler.

2.

REMEMBER, THE JOURNEY OF A THOUSAND MILES BEGINS WITH A SINGLE STEP

I can vividly remember the first sentence I ever wrote in my very first book! Had I not written that first sentence, I wouldn't have finished that first book, or the second, and so on. And so it goes. Every journey begins with a single step. But you *must* take that first step.

Sometimes when you consider taking on a new venture, the task can seem overwhelming. It feels as though you'll never be able to arrive at your final destination, as if the first step isn't going to help.

The trick to success sounds very simplistic, because it *is* very simple: just begin. Take a single step, followed by another, and then another. Don't look too far out into the future, and don't look too far back, either.

I often hear people telling me about the book they are *going* to write, the business they are *going* to start, or the charity they are *planning* to help. But in many instances, these plans and dreams keep getting put off until "the conditions are right." In almost all cases, the conditions you are waiting for will *not* be significantly different next week or next year. Don't worry that the conditions have to be perfect. The truth is, you are *still* going to have to take that first step!

3.

DARE TO BE HAPPY

Many people don't allow themselves the luxury of being enthusiastic, lighthearted, inspired, relaxed, or happy—especially at work. To me, this is a very unfortunate form of self-denial. The logic goes something like this: If they look happy, others might assume they are satisfied with the status quo and therefore lack the necessary motivation to excel in their work or go the extra mile. They certainly couldn't survive in a competitive environment.

I'm hired to speak to corporations around the country on stress reduction and happier living. On a number of occasions, the person who invited me to speak has asked me, in a nervous tone, if my talk would help the employees become *so* happy that they would "lose their edge." I'm not kidding!

In reality, it's nonsense to believe that a relaxed, happy person lacks motivation. On the contrary, happy people are almost always the ones who love what they do. It's been shown again and again that people who love what they do are highly motivated by their own enthusiasm to continually better themselves and their performance.

If you dare to be happy, your life will begin to change immediately. Your life and your work will take on greater significance and will be experienced as an extraordinary adventure.

4.

LEARN TO LAUGH AT YOURSELF

Almost nothing immunizes you from day-to-day frustration more than a healthy sense of humor—particularly the ability to laugh at yourself. If you are unable to laugh at yourself, you're in for a long, bumpy ride.

It's quite remarkable to observe what happens to a potentially heated interaction when someone is able to keep their sense of humor. In most cases, the situation is diffused and simply melts away. For example, my wife and I were sharing time with another couple when the woman made a slightly snide comment to her husband. Specifically, she said, "You talk too much." He laughed to himself and said, very gently, "You're right, I sure can dominate a conversation." More than his words, his ability to see a grain of truth in his wife's statement, to remain humble, and to be willing to chuckle at his own tendency resolved the situation before it had a chance to gain any momentum.

By laughing at yourself, not taking yourself so seriously, you will become much easier to be around. In the end, you will have created a more nourishing and safer environment for your partner, family, and friends, and your relationships will be more loving and a heck of lot more fun.

5.

LEARN THE MAGIC OF NONATTACHMENT

Without realizing it, many of us confuse nonattachment with not caring. In actuality, the two are completely different. Not caring suggests apathy: "I couldn't care less. It doesn't matter to me." Nonattachment, on the other hand, means: "I'll do everything possible, I'll put the odds in my favor, I'll work hard and concentrate. I'll do my best to succeed. *But* if I don't, that's okay, too."

Being attached to an outcome, holding on, takes an enormous amount of energy, not only during an effort but often after an effort is complete, after you've failed, been let down, or were dealt a bad hand.

Being nonattached, however, creates emotional freedom. It means holding on tightly but letting go lightly. It suggests trying hard, really caring, but at the same time being completely willing to let go of the outcome.

Attachment creates fear that gets in your way: *What if I lose? What if the deal doesn't go through? What if I'm rejected? What if, what if, what if*... Everything rides on your success.

Nonattachment, on the other hand, works like magic. The act of *not* worrying helps you focus and stay on task. You know in your heart that, even if things don't work out the way you hope they will, everything will be all right. You'll be okay.

6.

LET IT GO ALREADY

One day I was driving in a car, listening to a radio call-in talk show. In less than half an hour, three people called in to complain about something minor their spouse had done, or in one case "may have done," over a year ago.

I felt like yelling, "Let it go already!" Relationships can be challenging enough without the added burden of keeping past issues alive and vibrant in your mind. It's helpful to remind yourself of what happens to your own capacity to love, forgive, and grow when you are consumed with the past. Usually, when your head is filled with reminders of past issues and problems, you are filled with fear, suspicion, and frustration. Your frustration will usually spill over, and you'll probably end up being upset about all sorts of "small stuff."

The truth is, we all make mistakes, act less than perfect, and have at least occasional errors in judgment. The ideal environment to get through these things, however, is an environment of forgiveness and nonjudgment.

So, if you're carrying around or still holding on to issues from your past, it may be time to simply let them go. Make the decision to forgive, forget, and move on. You'll be rewarded with a richer, more open, honest, and far more loving and nourishing relationship.

7.

MAKE PEACE WITH IMPERFECTION

I've yet to meet an absolute perfectionist whose life was filled with inner peace. The need for perfection and the desire for inner tranquility conflict with each other. Whenever we are attached to having something a certain way, better than it already is, we are, almost by definition, engaged in a losing battle.

Whether it's related to ourselves—a disorganized closet, a scratch on the car, an imperfect accomplishment—or someone else's "imperfections"—the way someone looks, behaves, or lives their life—the very act of focusing on imperfection pulls us away from our goal of being kind and gentle. This strategy has nothing to do with ceasing to do your very best, but rather with recognizing when you are overly attached and focused on what's wrong with life. It's about realizing that while there's always a better way to do something, this doesn't mean that you can't enjoy and appreciate the way things already are.

The solution here is to catch yourself when you fall into your habit of insisting that things should be other than they are. Gently remind yourself that life is okay the way it is, right now. In the absence of your judgment, everything would be fine. As you begin to eliminate your need for perfection in all areas of your life, you'll begin to discover the perfection in life itself.

8.

CONSIDER THAT THE GRASS PROBABLY *ISN'T* GREENER

We live in what might be called the "trade up" era. We trade smaller homes for bigger ones, older cars for newer. We want better jobs, more income, a bigger retirement plan, and better experiences. We want better bodies and to belong to the best gym. Popular mottos include "New and improved" and "Out with the old and in with the new." We want, we want, we want. Always more. Something else is always going to be better.

It's helpful to realize and admit that often the fantasy of something different is a lot better than the reality of something different. We've met men and women who have left their spouses for someone else—someone younger or better looking, or someone who gave them more attention or who had more money—or whatever. Without exception, the fantasy was better than the reality.

When you find yourself thinking in these terms—always looking to "trade up" in whatever area of your life—try something a little different. Instead of distracting yourself with thoughts of what or who would be better, see if you can find a way to make the relationship you're already in be as good as it can be. Appreciate what you have now, and you'll probably discover that the grass isn't always greener.

9.

BECOME A STRESS-STOPPER

Often we feel compelled to share the details of our stressful thoughts with others around us, thereby encouraging them to get caught up in our dramas or to focus on other things they perceive to be stressful. We think about, commiserate, and emphasize the negative. It's hard to imagine anything less effective than an entire group of people upset, irritated, and stressed out!

When you make the conscious decision to become a stress-stopper, you'll find yourself nipping tons of stress—especially stress that is "small stuff"—in the bud. Your refusal to "spread the virus" not only prevents stress from escalating around you, but actually reinforces to you that many of the things we get all worked up about are, in the scheme of things, pretty irrelevant.

I was once driving to the airport with Kris and the kids, certain we were going to miss our flight. I must have mentioned my pessimistic prediction more than a dozen times. When we ended up making the flight, I realized how silly it had been to draw them into it—there was no upside; only downside.

Obviously, there are times when it's necessary or useful to share our stress with others. Yet if you're honest about it, I think you'll find that much of the time it's better and ultimately more effective to be a stress-stopper rather than a stress-spreader.

10.

LET GO OF THE IDEA THAT GENTLE, RELAXED PEOPLE CAN'T BE SUPERACHIEVERS

One of the major reasons so many of us remain hurried, frightened, and competitive, and continue to live life as if it were one giant emergency, is our fear that if we were to become more peaceful and loving, we would suddenly stop achieving our goals. We would become lazy and apathetic.

You can put this fear to rest by realizing that the opposite is actually true. Fearful, frantic thinking takes an enormous amount of energy and drains the creativity and motivation from our lives. When you are fearful or frantic, you literally immobilize yourself from your greatest potential, not to mention enjoyment. Any success that you do have is despite your fear, not because of it.

I have had the good fortune to surround myself with some very relaxed, peaceful, and loving people. Some of these people are best-selling authors, loving parents, counselors, computer experts, and chief executive officers. All of them are fulfilled in what they do and are very proficient at their given skills.

I have learned the important lesson: When you have what you want (inner peace), you are less distracted by your wants, needs, desires, and concerns. It's thus easier to concentrate, focus, achieve your goals, and to give back to others.

11.

BECOME LESS CONTROLLING

When I talk about being "controlling," I'm referring to unhealthy attempts to manipulate the behavior of others, having the need to control your environment, insisting on having things be "just so" in order to feel secure. To be controlling means you are preoccupied with the actions of others and how those actions affect you.

One of the most extreme examples of controlling behavior I've heard of involved, of all things, paper clips! A lawyer at a top-flight law firm had a penchant for certain things to be done in certain ways. This fellow liked to use copper-colored paper clips instead of the silver ones his firm provided (what could be more important than that?). So every week he had his secretary buy him his own private supply (and didn't even reimburse her). If something came to his desk with the wrong kind of clip, he'd fly into a rage. He became known in the office as "the paper clip king." Ultimately, his controlling behavior turned off one too many of his clients, and he was let go from the firm.

This is a very unusual and extreme example; yet if you examine your own behavior, you may find areas that you are trying to control that are futile or just plain silly. I encourage you to take a look.

12.

BE KIND FIRST (KRIS)

Above all else, adopt an attitude of kindness. Make it your highest priority to practice it every day. Start at home—in your relationships. Kindness is one of the primary ingredients in nourishing a warm feeling between people.

Being genuinely kind is not about smiling when you don't feel like it or acting cheerful when you're low. Rather, it's about treating your partner (and everyone else) the way you would like to be treated. It's been said many times that, in life, we teach people how to treat us. The best way to teach others (including our partner) that we would like to be treated with kindness is by offering our kindness first.

You start with the little things—listening from the heart and being respectful and thoughtful. Being kind means asking permission, when appropriate, and saying "I'm sorry" when you're wrong or when you make a mistake.

People are like mirrors of one another. For the most part, we get back that which we put out. The next time the person you love is having a bad day, try something a little different. Look them in the eye with a smile that says, "It's okay," and "I love you all the time, even when you're low." Chances are, if you do, you'll get a smile in return.

13.

BE AWARE OF THE SNOWBALL EFFECT OF YOUR THINKING

A powerful technique for becoming more peaceful is to be aware of how quickly your negative and insecure thinking can spiral out of control. Have you ever noticed how uptight you feel when you're caught up in your thinking? The more absorbed you get in the details of whatever is upsetting you, the worse you feel. One thought leads to another until you become incredibly agitated.

For example, you might wake up in the middle of the night and remember a phone call you need to make. Rather than feeling relieved that you remembered, you start thinking about everything else you have to do tomorrow. Pretty soon you think to yourself, "I can't believe how busy I am. Whose life is this anyway?" and on and on. For many people, there's no limit to how long this type of "thought attack" can go on.

The solution is to notice what's happening in your head before your thoughts have a chance to build any momentum. The sooner you catch yourself in the act of snowballing, the easier it is to stop. Say to yourself, "Whew, there I go again," and consciously nip it in the bud. Try this simple little exercise the next time you begin to obsess or worry. You'll be amazed at how effective it can be.

14.

FILL YOUR LIFE WITH OPPORTUNITIES TO EXPRESS LOVE

The feeling of love is contagious. When your heart is open and you're busy sharing your love with others, you draw more love in your direction.

There are countless ways to express love and to receive love. Anything you enjoy, that nurtures your spirit in a loving way, that allows you to share your love with something or someone else, has the potential to fill your heart with love. One of the most loving times in my life was when I was volunteering as a "big brother" for the Big Brothers of America organization. The experience changed my life, and my guess is that it wasn't a coincidence that I met Kris shortly thereafter.

When we're only looking to be loved, it's easy to forget how wonderful it is to give love. Yet when we discover new ways to share our love, an almost magical transformation takes place in our lives. We become more interested in others, more inclusive, and wiser. It almost seems like a law of nature—the more ways we discover to be loving, the more we find ourselves surrounded by the feeling of love.

Whatever your circumstances, dreams, or preferences, filling your life with opportunities to express your love is always a good idea.

15.

EXPERIENCE RELAXED PASSION

Passion takes different forms. It can be the feeling of being driven to success, of rolling up your sleeves, or working long hours. This "hyper" passion can be very exciting. The problem with it, though, is that it drains your energy. It's generated from external sources, from tight deadlines and big deals. Because of the external nature of this type of passion, a tint of fear always goes along with it: "I love this as long as everything works out well."

Another, calmer type of passion is what I call relaxed passion. This is a contained, "time-release" feeling that permeates everything you do. It brings joy and great success to virtually anything. Rather than being frenetic, this feeling is more like exhilaration and enthusiasm. It's a much calmer version of excitement, without the worry: "I love this simply because I'm absorbed in what I'm doing."

The way to bring forth this type of passion is to learn to keep your attention fully in the present moment. Try to do only one thing at any given moment and give that "one thing" your full and complete attention.

Almost anything we do is a potential source of relaxed passion. And it comes from our own attention, our own thinking. You can bring passion back into your life by simply being more oriented in the present moment.

16.

REMEMBER TO APPRECIATE THE PEOPLE YOU WORK WITH

One of the most consistent complaints of working people in virtually all industries is that they either feel completely unappreciated or, at the very least, underappreciated.

People need and deserve to feel appreciated. People who feel appreciated are happier, less stressed, and more loyal than those who feel taken for granted. Overall, they are harder workers and are excellent team players. Perhaps most of all, people who feel unappreciated have a tendency to sweat the small stuff.

Even if someone is "just doing her job," it's critical that she feels appreciated. My suggestion is to go out of your way to make sure those you work with know that you genuinely appreciate them. Praise often. Dish out compliments. If it's at all possible and appropriate, send a card, e-mail, or handwritten note. Make a phone call or, even better, look the person in the eye and tell them how much you appreciate them.

For example, even if it's the job of the mailroom guy to bring your mail, thank him when he drops it off. Thank the person at the copy shop for copying your papers. Yes, it's "her job"—so what?

I can't think of very many things that feel better than offering genuine appreciation toward those you work with.

17.

DEVELOP YOUR COMPASSION

Nothing helps us build our perspective more than developing compassion for others. Compassion is a sympathetic feeling. It involves the willingness to put yourself in someone else's shoes, to take the focus off yourself and to imagine what it's like to be in someone else's predicament, and simultaneously, to feel love for that person.

Compassion is something you can develop with practice. It involves two things: intention and action. Intention simply means you remember to open your heart to others; you expand what and who matters, from yourself to other people. Action is simply the "what you do about it." You might donate a little money or time (or both) on a regular basis to a cause near to your heart. Or perhaps you'll offer a beautiful smile and genuine "hello" to the people you meet on the street. It's not so important what you do, just that you do something.

When you take time, often, to reflect on the miracle of life—the miracle that you are even able to read this book—the gift of sight, of love, and all the rest, it can help to remind you that many of the things that you think of as "big stuff" are really just "small stuff" that you are turning into big stuff.

18.

LOOK FOR THE GIFTS

The human mind is an amazing thing in that, whatever it's looking for, it tends to find. So, if you're looking for ugliness, you'll have no trouble finding it. If you're looking for cruelty, again, you'll find plenty of evidence of that, too. And if you're looking for beauty, you'll be able to find that, as well.

Imagine that your partner is offered a job in a different part of the country. This could be seen as a major hassle or even a tragedy. If you focus on this aspect of it and express this position, you'll probably feel bad or be seen as an unsupportive spouse. If you were looking for a gift, however, it might be seen as an ideal chance to demonstrate how supportive you can be, or as an opportunity to begin a new adventure together.

When you're looking for the gifts in a situation, you'll almost always be able to find something positive to focus on. When this becomes your normal way of perceiving things, you'll find that it's almost impossible to get too upset over daily things, especially "small stuff."

19.

DO GOOD WHILE DOING WELL

People everywhere are looking for, and finding, ways to combine business with good works.

I was discussing this topic at a book signing when a somewhat cynical gentleman commented, "Easy for you to say." Before I even had a chance to respond, a little boy, no more than ten years old, stood up and said, "Do you want to know what I do?" "Sure," I said. "We'd all love to hear." "I keep track of my sales. After every hundred cups of lemonade I sell, I donate a whole pitcher to the retirement home down the street." The crowd loved it! Can you imagine how hard it would be to *not* buy lemonade from this young man?

If a ten-year-old's lemonade stand can be a vehicle to help others, why can't the rest of us contribute? You can donate a portion of your money, time, or energy. Whether you formalize it or not, there are thousands of ways to be helpful. I've found that people who consciously set out to be helpful to others are far less likely to sweat the small stuff.

I often wonder what kind of world we'd live in if everyone looked at their work as an opportunity to be of help. If each of us does our own little part, we just may find out someday.

20.

ELIMINATE THE RAT RACE MENTALITY

I often hear people conversing about being stuck "in the rat race" as if they were discussing the weather—in a very casual, matter-of-fact manner. The assumption seems to be that it's inevitable.

So much of our daily work life exists in our own mind, dependent upon what aspects we focus on and how we characterize our experience. In other words, when we describe our day, we say, "It was awful. I was stuck in horrible traffic with millions of other angry people. I spent my day in boring meetings. There were arguments and almost constant conflict to deal with. What a bunch of jerks!"

The identical day might be thought of differently. You might describe it like this: "I drove to work and spent much of my day meeting with people. It was a challenge, but I did my best to stay on top of it. The art of my work is bringing together people who, on the surface, don't seem to be able to get along very well. It's a good thing I'm there to help."

Can you feel the difference? And it's not a matter of one description being "realistic and accurate" and the other being wishful thinking. Both are absolutely accurate. It all depends on the well-being of the person doing the thinking.

21.

ALLOW TIME FOR TRANSITIONS

There are many periods of transition in life. I've found that the most graceful way to move through these transitions is to make allowances for them by allowing plenty of time. When you make the assumption that a transition is going to take time, it seems to take the urgency, as well as much of the frustration, out of the picture. It allows you the time to settle in.

Two of my dearest friends moved to a new location. They had a young child, were unfamiliar with the new city, and initially had no friends. Rather than become despondent or frightened, they decided to embrace the philosophy of allowing time for their transition. They decided they wouldn't expect to feel settled for at least a year. Then, with each new friend they met and each positive experience they had, they were delighted and grateful. They eased into their new lives and are now happier than ever before.

Transitions are like speed bumps: You need to slow down while approaching them. Rather than expecting your life to remain the same, or trying to re-create the life you are most familiar with, try to be open and accepting to change. If you allow for plenty of time for your transitions, you will, like a dancer, gracefully adjust to the next step in the process.

22.

REMIND YOURSELF THAT WHEN YOU DIE, YOUR INBOX WON'T BE EMPTY

So many of us live our lives as if the secret purpose is to somehow get everything done. We stay up late, get up early, avoid having fun, and keep our loved ones waiting. We convince ourselves that once we get through our to-do list, we'll be calm, relaxed, and happy. But in reality, this rarely happens. As items are checked off, new ones simply replace them.

The nature of your inbox is that it's *meant* to have items to be completed in it—it's not meant to be empty. There will always be e-mails to send, projects to complete, and work to be done.

Regardless of who you are or what you do, however, remember that nothing is more important than your own sense of happiness and inner peace and that of your loved ones. In reality, almost everything can wait. Very little in our work lives truly falls into the "emergency" category. It will all get done in due time.

When you die, there will still be unfinished business to take care of. And you know what? Someone else will do it for you! Don't waste any more precious moments of your life regretting the inevitable.

23.

PUT A POSITIVE SPIN ON IT

In politics, the term *spin* has taken on a negative connotation. In personal relationships, however, it's a far different story. The idea of putting a positive spin on the events, circumstances, and challenges of your relationships can become one of the most important habits you can incorporate into your life.

There's a story of two bricklayers who have identical jobs. Someone asks the first man, "What is it that you do?" He answers bitterly: "I sit here every day laying one stupid brick on top of another." The man asks the other bricklayer the same question. He says in a confident, upbeat manner, "I am a craftsman. I help build all the beautiful buildings you see around you. Without my contribution, none of this would be here." Both men are right!

It's easy to see that you can take almost any situation and look at it in two ways. You can look for what's in it for you, any hidden gifts that might be found, and for what you can learn from it. Or you can see difficulties and hassles as simply more evidence that life is hard and unfair.

Obviously, reading this strategy doesn't mean you'll always be able to look at events from a more positive perspective (we can't either), but it's sure comforting to know that the possibility exists.

24.

DON'T DEAL WITH PROBLEMS, TRANSCEND THEM

When I suggest that clients *not* work on problems, they often appear irritated, as if I'm telling them not to bathe or brush their teeth! This is because most people assume that the only way to solve problems is to work on, or struggle, with them. I have found, however, that focusing on problems is one of the key ways of keeping them alive—as well as preventing you from moving past them. I promise that there is a way to get from where you are to where you want to be *without* focusing on problems.

The thoughts we have around our various issues—personal and professional—create and trigger emotional reactions. What usually happens is that we spend our time and energy dealing with these reactions instead of the actual issue. Simply put, when we are frightened, angry, or impatient, we lose our bearings and get in our own way.

The alternative to dealing head-on with problems is to clear your mind instead of filling it with painful, confusing details. Quiet down, reflect, and listen. Allow your wisdom, that softer part of your thinking, to surface. More often than not, seemingly out of nowhere, you will have an insight, an answer to your problem. Nevertheless, the less you worry about your problems, the easier they will be to solve!

25.

DON'T INTERRUPT OTHERS OR FINISH THEIR SENTENCES

It wasn't until a few years ago that I realized how often I interrupted others and finished their sentences. Shortly thereafter, I also realized how destructive this habit was, not only to the respect and love I received from others but also for the tremendous amount of energy it takes to try to be in two heads at once! Think about it for a moment. When you interrupt someone or finish their sentence, you have to keep track not only of your own thoughts but those of the person you are interrupting as well. This tendency encourages both parties to speed up their speech and their thinking. This, in turn, makes both people nervous, irritable, and annoyed. It's downright exhausting.

Once you begin noticing yourself interrupting others, you'll see that this insidious tendency is nothing more than an innocent habit that has become invisible to you. This is good news because it means that all you really have to do is to begin catching yourself when you forget. Remind yourself to be patient and wait. The people you communicate with will feel much more relaxed around you when they feel heard and listened to. You'll also notice how much more relaxed you'll feel when you stop interrupting others.

26.

CONSIDER THE POSSIBILITY THAT IF IT SOUNDS TOO GOOD TO BE TRUE, IT MIGHT NOT BE

The adage "If it sounds too good to be true, it probably is" isn't always correct. In fact, the suspicion, cynicism, and doubt that are inherent in this belief can and do keep people from taking advantage of excellent opportunities.

Cynicism contradicts abundance. Cynics, critics, and doubters are clouded by their own destructive, self-defeating filters that say things like "That can't work," "That's impossible," or "It's too good to be true."

I was lucky enough to hear about a great stock from a good friend of mine. He told me and a few others. Unfortunately for my other friends, they instantly dismissed the suggestion. I've learned, however, to keep an open mind. I did my research and decided to buy some shares. Lo and behold, the stock doubled in less than a month. Lucky? Of course. But had I not been open-minded, I wouldn't have been in a position to be lucky!

If you think something is too good to be true, you'll be very hesitant to take a careful look at it, and you'll dismiss it as being superficial or too risky. Often, there are great deals and wonderful opportunities that come your way. But to take advantage of them, you must be open, willing to take a look, and ready to learn something new or try something different.

27.

SET A GOOD EXAMPLE (KRIS)

We've all heard it said that you can't change other people. It's a strange thing, though. We all seem to find things that we'd like to change, don't we? However, setting a good example yourself is the best way to influence change in your loved ones.

My friend Barbara devoted a great part of her life to health and fitness. There came a time a few years ago that it became necessary, for health reasons, for her husband, Don, to adopt a new, drastically different lifestyle.

Barbara realized that the only way Don would adhere to the strict vegetarian diet ordered by his doctor was if she adopted it too, which is exactly what she did. Rather than badger him about it, she decided to set the good example. Today, both Barbara and Don are visions of excellent health.

This strategy also pertains to happiness. Over the years, I have watched Richard gracefully move through his high and low moods; he has taught me, by example, to do the same. Rather than lecture me, he simply shows me.

Mental health, loving energy, and good habits are contagious. If there's something in your loved ones you'd like to see change, take stock of yourself first. Set the example by the way you live, and eventually they may come around, too.

28.

HAVE SOME "NO E-MAIL" TIME AT WORK

If you're like me, e-mail is a mixed bag of goods. On one hand, it's a lifesaver and obviously critical to most people. Without it, work would be impossible. On the other hand, depending on what you do for a living, the e-mail can be one of the most distracting and stressful aspects of your work.

In my office, if I didn't have any "no e-mail" time, I would be dealing with e-mail close to 100 percent of the day. If I didn't have protective policies in place, I'd have very little time to write or work on other projects. I suspect the same may be true for many of you.

You can set this strategy in place in many different ways. I have certain times of the day when I turn off notifications and don't reply. This gives me some time to focus—without distraction—on what's most relevant to my work.

Let's face it. The work world is not going to accommodate us with fewer e-mails to respond to. I've found that I can get twice, even three times the amount of concentrated work done when I'm not distracted by e-mail. Then, with all the time I have saved, I can almost always reply when everything else has been done.

29.

DO SOMETHING NICE FOR SOMEONE ELSE AND DON'T TELL *ANYONE* ABOUT IT

While many of us frequently do nice things for others, we are almost certain to mention our acts of kindness to someone else, secretly seeking their approval.

When we share our own niceness or generosity with someone else, it makes us feel like we are thoughtful people, and it reminds us of how nice we are and how deserving we are of kindness.

While all acts of kindness are inherently wonderful, there is something even more magical about doing something thoughtful but mentioning it to no one, ever. You always feel good when you give to others. Rather than diluting the positive feelings by telling others about your own kindness, by keeping it to yourself you get to retain *all* the positive feelings.

It's really true that one should give for the sake of giving, not to receive something in return. This is precisely what you are doing when you don't mention your kindness to others—your rewards are the warm feelings that come from the act of giving. The next time you do something really nice for someone else, keep it to yourself and revel in the abundant joy of giving.

30.

DON'T DRAMATIZE THE DEADLINES

Have you ever stopped to think about how much mental and emotional emphasis we put on our deadlines? And have you ever wondered what negative consequences are attached to such emphasis?

Recently, I overheard two coworkers talking in the office. They were complaining about the unfair tight deadline they were on. Apparently, they had less than two hours to complete a report. I sat there, listening in amazement, as the two of them spent almost an entire hour complaining about how ridiculous the deadline was. Finally, one of them said in a frantic tone, "God, we'd better get started. It's due in an hour."

It's been my experience that complaining about deadlines—even if the complaints are justified—takes an enormous amount of mental energy and, more important to deadlines, time! The added obsessive thinking about the deadline creates its own internal anxiety.

I know that deadlines can create quite a bit of stress and that sometimes it doesn't seem fair. See if you can notice how often you tend to worry, fret, or complain about deadlines. Then, try to catch yourself in the act of doing so. When you do, gently remind yourself that your energy would be better spent elsewhere.

31.

START THE DAY WITH LOVE, LIVE THE DAY WITH LOVE, END THE DAY WITH LOVE

The wisdom of this strategy is quite simple. The idea is to remind yourself frequently, throughout the day, of the importance of living your life with *love* as your absolute top priority. Something magical happens to your life when nothing is seen as more important than love. Our day-to-day living begins to take on an extraordinary quality and we begin to experience what's truly most important in life.

"Start the day with love" means that when you wake up, you open your heart and remind yourself of your intent to be loving in every aspect of your life. "Live the day with love" means that your choices and actions stem from your decision to be loving, patient, kind, and gentle. It means you keep things in perspective and try *not* to take things personally or blow things out of proportion. "End the day with love" means that you take a moment at the close of your day to reflect and be grateful. You might look back on your day and review how closely your *goal* of living with love matched with your actions and choices. You do this not to keep score, but simply to experience the peace associated with loving intent and to see areas where you might act even more loving tomorrow.

32.

BECOME LESS REACTIVE AND MORE RESPONSIVE

In personal and professional life, we have essentially two psychological modes that we are in most of the time: reactive and responsive.

The reactive mode is the one that feels stressful. In it, we feel pressured, lose perspective, and take things personally. Needless to say, our judgment and decision-making capacity is severely impaired when we are in a reactive state of mind. We make quick decisions that we often regret. We annoy other people and bring out the worst in them.

The responsive mode, on the other hand, is our most relaxed state of mind. Being responsive suggests that we have our bearings. We see the bigger picture and take things less personally. Rather than being rigid and stubborn, we are flexible and calm. In the responsive mode, we are at our best.

Simply becoming aware of the different dynamics of your mind will open the door to tremendous changes in your life. You'll begin to notice when you fall into a reactive state of mind. You'll feel your own impatience. When this happens, simply acknowledge your mind-set. You'll discover, as you notice and acknowledge your own reactivity, coupled with your understanding that, in all cases, it pays to be more responsive, you'll quickly come out of a reactive mode and fall into a more responsive state of mind.

33.

LET OTHERS HAVE THE GLORY

There is something magical that happens to the human spirit, a sense of calm that comes over you, when you cease needing all the attention directed toward yourself and instead allow others to have the glory.

Our need for excessive attention is that ego-centered part of us that says, "Look at me. I'm special. My story is more interesting than yours." The ego is that part of us that wants to be seen, heard, respected, and considered special, often at the expense of someone else.

The next time someone tells you a story or shares an accomplishment with you, notice your tendency to say something about yourself in response.

Although it's a difficult habit to break, it's not only enjoyable but actually peaceful to have the quiet confidence to be able to surrender your need for attention and instead share in the joy of someone else's glory. Just say, "That's wonderful," or "Please tell me more," and leave it at that. The person you are speaking with will have so much more fun, and, because you are so much more "present" and are listening so carefully, they won't feel in competition with you.

Obviously, there are many times when it's absolutely appropriate to exchange experiences back and forth and to share in the glory and attention rather than giving it all away.

34.

WORK ON "KNOWING" INSTEAD OF "BELIEVING"

When you *believe* something, it's usually because someone told you to—your parents, an instructor, a friend, a colleague, a partner, a boss. You were influenced, often in a positive way, by what you were told. Consequently, your belief system was formed in some measurable way.

Knowing, on the other hand, is intrinsic in nature. When you know something, you feel it. You may not always be able to explain or articulate how or why, but something within you is providing you with needed answers and guiding you in a direction.

For example, I always knew that I would be a teacher of some kind. This is difficult to explain because I nearly flunked high school English and actually fainted while public speaking! Perhaps the *only* thing I did right was listen to my inner voice. It took many years to find my path, but knowing is always more powerful than believing.

All of us have things that we know to be true about ourselves—dreams that we have, gifts we wish to share, unique talents we want to pursue. But all too often our beliefs convince us to ignore our knowing. The moment you decide that what you *know* is more important than what you have been taught to *believe*, you will be on the right path.

35.

AVOID CORPORATE BRAGGING

In my work as a coach and speaker, I've noticed a destructive tendency that I call "corporate bragging."

Corporate bragging is sharing with others how incredibly busy you are and how very hard you work—not just in passing, but rather as a central, focal point of conversation. It's almost as though we wear a badge of honor for being a person who is completely overwhelmed, deprived of sleep, and who has little, if any, personal life. I've heard people brag about not having time to go out on dates or about being so busy and frantic that they've forgotten to eat.

Although "corporate bragging" is a catchy phrase, the tendency itself is certainly not limited to people working in the corporate world.

The problem is that bragging about how busy you are reinforces to yourself how stressed out you are. It keeps you overly focused on the most negative aspects of your work. It becomes a self-fulfilling prophecy, keeping you caught up in your own business. Not to mention, it's not very interesting to hear about how busy or overwhelmed you are.

So, no matter how you look at it, corporate bragging does no good. If you're too busy, you either need to cut back or catch up. But talking about it to others only exacerbates your stress and makes you a less interesting person.

36.

BE AWARE OF WHAT YOU DON'T KNOW AND WHAT YOU'RE NOT GOOD AT

My father used to tell me as he read my poorly written essays in school, "Richard, it's not important that you're not a great speller. It's really important, however, that you know that you're not a good speller. That way, when in doubt, you can use the dictionary." Boy, was he right!

The same idea applies to virtually everything. In my work, for example, it's not critical that I'm an expert editor as long as I know my own weaknesses and limitations. I can hire someone to fill in where I'm weak. The only time there would be a problem is if I didn't know that I wasn't good at something or if I was unwilling to admit it.

Chances are you're probably really good at certain things and really bad at others. So what? Why should you frustrate yourself and waste your time doing those things you struggle with? This doesn't mean you can't learn new skills or improve existing ones. It merely suggests that you spend the bulk of your time doing whatever it is you do best.

What if you could spend an extra two or three hours a day focusing on that which you truly love and are genuinely good at? You'll never know for sure until you try!

37.

AVOID THE "I'VE HAD A REALLY HARD DAY" HABIT

One of my family's favorite songs is Shania Twain's "Honey, I'm Home." The kids in particular love to sing along in the backseat. In this upbeat, funny song, Twain sings about what a "hard day" she has had. She goes into tremendous detail about everything that went wrong. One thing after another. Everything that could have possibly gone wrong did. Anyone who has ever had a horrible day can relate.

While I'm the first to admit that there are times when a long complaining session feels really good or even necessary and cleansing, the truth is, there isn't a correlation between reviewing negative events and a positive, uplifted feeling. It's actually the other way around.

Again, no one is denying that life can be hard and that certain days are particularly difficult. Every once in a while, all of us need a listening ear, and upon occasion it's perfectly okay and healthy to vent. But try to avoid making the negative events of your day the primary topic of your evening conversation. When you nip this habit in the bud, you'll become aware of far more of what's good in life, and this joy will spread to your relationships.

38.

LEARN TO LIVE IN THE PRESENT MOMENT

To a large degree, the measure of our peace of mind is determined by how much we are able to live in the present moment. Regardless of what happened yesterday or last year, and what may or may not happen tomorrow, the present moment is where you are—always!

Without question, many of us have mastered the neurotic art of spending much of our lives worrying about a variety of things—all at once. We allow past problems and future concerns to dominate our present moments, and end up anxious, frustrated, depressed, and hopeless. On the flip side, we also postpone our gratification, our stated priorities, and our happiness, often convincing ourselves that "someday" will be better than today. Either way, we miss out on life.

When our attention is in the present moment, we push fear from our minds. Practice keeping your attention on the here and now. Your efforts will pay great dividends.

39.

REDUCE YOUR SELF-INDUCED STRESS

An insightful colleague of mine had a terrific idea for a T-shirt. He was going to call it something like "The Shirt to Take Away Your Stress" and offer a 100 percent guarantee that while you were wearing the shirt, you would never feel any stress—other than the stress you create in your own head!

Obviously, his premise was that all of your stress originates from the way that you think, so he would never have to return any money. I wouldn't go quite that far, but his point is well taken.

While there are some situations that are inherently stressful, it's clear that a significant percentage of the stress we feel does indeed originate from within us—from the way we think and hold on to things. The hardest part of dealing with self-induced stress is to have the humility to admit that it is, indeed, self-induced. Once you see your part, however, you have the power to change.

Start by observing your thoughts. Are you practicing optimism, good mental health, and keeping your perspective? Or do you allow your thinking to get the best of you? Do you take your thinking too seriously? If so, this is the place to start. Remember, it's far easier to shift your thinking than it is to shift the ways of the world.

40.

THINK BEFORE YOU SPEAK

A dear friend had just returned home from a long bike ride. She was really excited because the time it took to complete the second half of the ride was less than the time it took to complete the first half. She had been training hard and was elated. As she walked in the front door, she shared her success with her husband. Without thinking, he blurted out, "The reason you were able to go faster on the way back is because there is more downhill."

Ouch! This tendency to speak without thinking comes out in many ways—sarcasm, put-downs, one-upping, correcting, or simply saying something a little mean. It usually happens when you're in a reactive state of mind, a little tired, overwhelmed, stressed, or frustrated.

A general rule of thumb is this: If you have even the slightest doubt about whether your upcoming response is appropriate, ask yourself the following two-part question: "Is my next comment going to add to this conversation? Is it going to bring us closer, or is it likely to drive us apart?"

This strategy is short and sweet. You can think of it as a heads-up, or a simple reminder that it's crucial that we pause for a moment when our loved one has finished speaking so that we can, in turn, think before we speak.

41.

BECOME AWARE OF THE PASSION FACTOR

Passion is a virtually unstoppable, attitudinal force that generates energy, creativity, and productivity. When you love what you do, it's difficult not to succeed. Your enthusiasm is obvious to everyone around you, and it is contagious.

Part of the process of creating passion in your life is choosing work that you truly love. Doing so requires conscious choice, which often takes a great deal of courage. It can be frightening to change career directions or to try something new, regardless of how much we may want to.

Fear is a powerful, highly destructive force, but if you take a careful look at most successful people, more often than not, they have faced very similar fears and conquered them. A client of mine once said, "I asked myself the question, 'Whose life is this anyway?' and when I couldn't answer the question, I knew I had to make a change."

It's important to ask yourself: "How safe is it, *really*, spending my time doing something I don't enjoy? How well can I perform a task I dread? How creative and original is my thinking?" The answers to each of these questions are clear: Without passion, your odds of success are minimal. When you discover what is truly nourishing to your soul, a joyful life is just around the corner.

42.

IMAGINE THAT EVERYONE IS ENLIGHTENED EXCEPT YOU

As the title suggests, the idea is to imagine that everyone you know and everyone you meet is perfectly enlightened. Everyone except you! The people you meet are all here to teach you something.

Your job is to try to determine what the people in your life are trying to teach you. You'll find that if you do this, you'll be far less annoyed, bothered, and frustrated by the actions and imperfections of other people. Get in the habit of approaching life in this manner and, if you do, you'll be glad you did.

Often, once you discover what someone is trying to teach you, it's easy to let go of your frustration. For example, suppose you're in the post office and the clerk is moving painfully slow. Ask yourself the question, "What is he trying to teach me?" Maybe you need to learn about compassion—how hard it would be to have a job that you don't like. Or perhaps you could learn a little more about being patient.

You may be surprised at how fun and easy this is. All you're really doing is changing your perception from "Why are they doing this?" to "What are they trying to teach me?"

43.

DON'T LET SUCCESS GO TO YOUR HEAD

There's an alarming trend taking place: People who have had some degree of good fortune and success tend to lose their humility and become at least slightly arrogant. This is very unfortunate for many reasons. First, and most obviously, no one really wants to be around someone who is arrogant or self-absorbed. Arrogance implies a lack of gratitude. The assumption is, "I did this all by myself; it's all about me."

In addition, when you allow success to go to your head, your stress levels skyrocket and your quality of life gradually disappears. People will stop liking you, and eventually, you'll stop liking yourself. In a way, it's ironic. Someone finally gets what they've always wanted—success—yet now they are rarely satisfied.

So, whether you've already made your fortune or are still working on it, try to see the absurdity and humor behind letting any type of success go to your head. Even if you've slipped in that direction, it's never too late to turn yourself around. You can have it all—tremendous success, good fortune, and a lifetime of abundance—and still be a thoughtful, kind, generous person. If you can do this, then you'll really have something, because not only will you be successful, you'll be happy as well!

44.

BANISH BOREDOM

Meetings can be one of the most dull parts of work life, but I've found two secrets to making virtually any meeting as interesting as it can possibly be. The first thing I do is use the meeting to practice being "present-moment oriented." In other words, I attempt to absorb myself in the meeting—not allowing my mind to wander. This deliberate attempt to be focused allows me to get as much value out of the experience as possible.

Since I've been doing this, I've found that the meetings I attend are far more interesting. Additional insights come to mind, and I feel as though I have more to offer. I've also noticed an increased sense of respect from others. It seems that when others in a meeting sense that you are truly listening, they want to listen to you as well. People are drawn to your energy and presence.

The second commitment I have made is to tell myself that I'm going to learn something new from each meeting. So, I listen intently to what is being said, trying to hear something I don't already know. In other words, rather than comparing what I'm hearing to what I already believe, I'm searching for new wisdom or a new way of doing something. I've found that when my intent is to learn, I almost always do learn.

45.

THINK GENTLE THOUGHTS

Being a generally optimistic person, I've always assumed that thinking positive thoughts was a major key to happiness. And while I still assume this to be the case, I've learned that perhaps even more powerful than thinking positive thoughts is learning to think gently.

An interesting exercise is to fill your mind with gentle, loving thoughts and then try to get irritated. My guess is that you won't be able to do it! The reason is, the qualities of a gentle mind are inconsistent with annoyance—the two are mutually exclusive. When your mind is gentle, your responses to ordinary events—especially small stuff—will tend to be compassionate. Typically, you'll be able to keep your sense of humor as well as your perspective. Rather than reacting harshly to the events of the day, you'll respond from a place of kindness. Simply put, the normal things that happen during the course of a day won't bug you quite as much and won't seem like such a big deal.

Gentle thoughts are those that reinforce the beauty of life and the privilege of being here. They range from thoughts of love and peace to those of forgiveness and generosity. They often include a hint of gratitude. Sometimes the simplest ideas are the most powerful.

46.

LET OTHERS BE "RIGHT" MOST OF THE TIME

One of the most important questions you can ever ask yourself is, "Do I want to be 'right' or do I want to be happy?" Many times, the two are mutually exclusive!

Being right and defending our positions takes an enormous amount of mental energy and often alienates us from the people in our lives. Needing to be right encourages others to become defensive, and puts pressure on us to keep defending.

We all want our positions to be respected and understood by others. Being listened to and heard is one of the greatest desires of the human heart. And those who learn to listen are the most loved and respected.

It's not that it's never appropriate to be right. Perhaps there are certain positions that you don't want to budge on, such as when you hear a racist comment. Here, it's important to speak your mind. Usually, however, it's just your ego creeping in and ruining an otherwise peaceful encounter.

A wonderful, heartfelt strategy for becoming more peaceful is to practice allowing others the joy of being right. Stop correcting. You'll discover the joy of participating in and witnessing other people's happiness, which is far more rewarding than a battle of egos. You don't have to sacrifice your deepest truths, but starting today, let others be "right" most of the time!

47.

BE WILLING TO CHANGE

In his wonderful book *Success Is No Accident*, Dr. Lair Ribeiro makes a statement that rings true to my ears and has been proven repeatedly throughout history. He says, "If you go on doing what you've always done, you'll go on getting what you've always got." What a powerful message! Sometimes, to create positive things in your life, you need to make some changes in the way you do things. The world isn't going to suddenly reward you by changing its conditions. Instead, *you* must alter the way you approach certain challenges.

I have met many people who are virtually unwilling to change, even when their current efforts aren't working. People are frightened of change. Maybe you're not the type of person who believes in asking friends and family for favors. And you might even be proud of this fact. Still, there are times when asking for help might be just what you need.

Take an inventory of your own stubbornness: Are there areas in your life where you do things a certain way simply because that's the way you've always done them? If you drop your fear and have the courage to be willing to change, my guess is that you won't have to go on much longer getting what you've always had.

48.

DON'T SWEAT YOUR CRITICS

No one is important enough, good enough, or well-intentioned enough to escape their share of criticism.

I asked a fellow author who is extremely calm and nonreactive how he handles bad reviews and criticism. He told me, "I always try to see if there is a grain of truth in what is being said. Quite honestly, there often is. In these instances, I try to learn what I can, and then let go of it. Very often my greatest growth comes directly after a dose of criticism. On the other hand, I've learned that if there's nothing to the criticism, it will simply fade away. The worst thing to do is take it personally and become defensive."

We will always run into people who have differing points of view and who see life very differently from the way we do. When this becomes okay with you, criticism won't have the same hold on you that it once did. Remember, the same thing that one person loves will irritate someone else.

When you make the decision to stop sweating your critics, your ego and self-image won't be hurt anymore, and your life will seem a great deal less stressful.

49.

BECOME MORE PATIENT

The quality of patience goes a long way toward your goal of creating a more peaceful and loving self. The more patient you are, the more accepting you will be of what is, rather than insisting that life be exactly as you would like it to be. Patience adds a dimension of ease and acceptance to your life.

Becoming more patient involves opening your heart to the present moment, even if you don't like it. In moments of tension, opening to the moment would mean catching yourself building a mental snowball and gently reminding yourself to relax. It might also be a good time to breathe, as well as an opportunity to remind yourself that this is "small stuff."

Patience also involves seeing the innocence in others. On many occasions while writing my early books, my young daughter would walk into my office and interrupt my work. I learned to see the innocence in her behavior rather than to focus on the potential implications of her interruption. I reminded myself *why* she was coming to see me—because she loves me.

I have found that, if you look deeply enough, you can almost always see the innocence in other people as well as in potentially frustrating situations.

50.

CREATE "PATIENCE PRACTICE" PERIODS

Patience is a quality of heart that can be greatly enhanced with deliberate practice. I've found that creating actual practice periods—periods of time that I set up in my mind to practice the art of patience—is a helpful tool.

You can start with as little as five minutes and build up your capacity for patience. Start by saying to yourself, "For the next five minutes I won't allow myself to be bothered by anything. I'll be patient." Your intention to be patient immediately strengthens your capacity for patience. You'll begin to see that you do, indeed, have the capacity to be patient, even for longer periods of time. Over time, you may even become a patient person.

With young children at home, I have many possibilities to practice the art of patience. For example, on a day when both girls are firing questions at me as I'm trying to work, I'll say to myself, "Now is a great time to be patient. For the next half hour I'm going to be as patient as possible (see, I've worked hard, I'm up to thirty minutes)!" All kidding aside, it really works.

Whether you're needing to deal with children, your boss, or a difficult situation—if you don't want to "sweat the small stuff," improving your patience level is a great way to start.

51.

CHOOSE PEACE OVER IRRITATION

To this day, I'm often surprised and delighted at the effectiveness of this simple yet powerful strategy. Every moment, it's as if we're at an emotional fork in the road. Something happens, followed by our choice either to react or to respond. Unfortunately, because we usually react so quickly and habitually, it often doesn't seem as though we have a choice. Our reactions seem to have a life of their own and occur almost instantly.

But when you look more carefully, you'll notice that you really do have a choice. Rather than reacting as you always do, you have the power and the ability to respond differently. And this is very important because, in the absence of your willingness to make this choice, you'll be frustrated each time something proves to be less than perfect.

This choice exists in virtually any situation. Dozens of times a day, things either go wrong or life turns out to be some way other than you would like it to be in that moment. And whether it's your partner acting in a way that you don't like or something else altogether, it's yet another chance to choose peace over irritation. This doesn't mean you're condoning bad behavior or that you don't care when things go wrong. It simply means that you've decided that being peaceful is the best way of being.

52.

EXPRESS YOUR GRATITUDE TOWARD OTHERS

There are very few sure things in life. But this is one of them: *As long as our expression of gratitude is genuine, other people love it and remember it. This not only makes them feel good, but it also encourages them to help us again and to encourage others to do the same.*

Most people love helping others, reaching out, lending a hand, offering assistance. The other side of the coin, however, is that people love to be acknowledged, admired, and thanked. People love to be thanked, not out of any selfish need but simply because it feels good to be acknowledged.

Many wonderful people have stepped forward to help me in my career and in my life. Whether I have asked for help or received it without request, I always try to remember to express my gratitude. None of us wants to be taken for granted. We all love to be thanked!

The next time you do something really nice or helpful for someone and they thank you, take note of how it makes you feel. There are many instances where you would help again without any thanks (parents know this!). I'll bet you'll find yourself even more willing to help someone who expresses their gratitude, which is, of course, also one of the keys to a joyful life.

53.

STOP ANTICIPATING TIREDNESS

Recently, I was on a flight from San Francisco to Chicago when I heard two people discussing how tired they were *going* to be—tomorrow and all week! They told stories of late nights, lack of sleep, uncomfortable hotel beds, and early morning meetings. They anticipated feeling exhausted, and I'm sure they were going to be correct in their assumption.

The problem with anticipating tiredness in this way, or in any way, is that it clearly reinforces the tiredness. It rivets your attention to the number of hours you are sleeping and how tired you are going to be.

Clearly, everyone needs a certain degree of rest. Many, if not most, of us don't get enough sleep. And if you're tired, the best possible solution would probably be to try to get more sleep. But in those instances when it's not possible to do so, the worst thing you can do, in my estimation, is to convince yourself, in advance, that you are going to be exhausted.

I've noticed this habit of anticipating tiredness creep into the conversations of many people (don't feel bad, I've done it plenty of times in the past). If you are someone who does this, see if you can avoid the tendency as much as possible. If you do, you may find yourself feeling less tired.

54.

WAIT FOR INSPIRATION

Ironically, it's often the case that the best use of our time is to do absolutely nothing—to not act, to simply wait for an answer. But in our speeded-up, frenetic culture, most of us panic if we aren't actively doing something, even if that "something" isn't wise, productive, or useful. Most of us are so busy, or at least looking busy, that we can't see or hear our own wisdom.

Built into our psyche is a wealth of wisdom. We all have innate common sense at our disposal that can provide us with solutions, inspiration, and guidance. The problem is, we must quiet down enough to hear it. We must wait for inspiration.

To access our innate health takes some humility and getting used to. We must be willing to admit that "we don't know what to do" at a given moment. We must learn to be a little patient; it's worth the wait. The simple act of admitting that you *don't know* an answer, at present, activates your inner wisdom and guidance. By simply being willing to wait for inspiration, you virtually guarantee that it will come—in most cases, rather quickly. The answers you receive, however, will surprise and delight you. Your thinking and instincts will rise to a new level.

55.

DISCOVER WHAT PART YOU ARE PLAYING

There are many characteristics that separate truly great relationships from all the others—a loving heart, thoughtfulness, generosity, a lack of jealousy, kindness, shared values, trust, integrity, to name just a few.

Here is another characteristic, however, to add to this illustrious list that is equally important, yet discussed and acknowledged far less often: the willingness and desire to acknowledge your own contributions to your problems. This willingness is so powerful that, combined with a loving heart, you'd be in pretty good shape if you did little else right.

You will identify solutions in a fraction of the time when you strive to see your part. Obviously this doesn't mean that all of the blame for every conflict lies with you, but owning your responsibility is a powerful way to invite change.

It's not always the case, but usually there are two sides to the issue—both parties contributing in some way to a problem. When neither person sees their own part, change is difficult, unlikely, or even impossible. However, when either person sees their contribution to a problem, a reasonable solution will usually surface. Give this strategy some thought, and your relationships will seem less confusing in no time.

56.

BE THE FIRST ONE TO ACT LOVING OR REACH OUT

So many of us hold on to little resentments that may have stemmed from an argument, a misunderstanding, the way we were raised, or some other painful event. Stubbornly, we wait for someone else to reach out to us.

An acquaintance of mine, whose health isn't very good, recently told me that she hasn't spoken to her son in almost three years. "Why not?" I asked. She said that she and her son had had a disagreement and that she wouldn't speak to him again unless he called first. When I suggested that she be the one to reach out, she resisted initially and said, "I can't do that. He's the one who should apologize." She was literally willing to die before reaching out to her only son. After a little gentle encouragement, however, she decided to be the first one to reach out. To her amazement, her son was grateful for her willingness to call and offered an apology of his own.

Whenever we hold on to our anger, we turn "small stuff" into really "big stuff" in our minds. We start to believe that our positions are more important than our happiness. They are not. The way to be happy is to let go, and reach out.

57.

USE THE POWER OF REFLECTION

Reflection is one of the most underused yet powerful tools for success. It is a passive way to pinpoint solutions with the least amount of effort or wasted energy. It's the opposite of "trying too hard," of forcing an answer. Reflection is more a matter of allowing an answer to unfold right before your eyes, often with little or no effort on your part.

One of the benefits of reflection is that it enables us to get our egos out of the way. In a quiet state of mind we are able to see things clearly, including our own contributions to problems and new ways of doing things. We can sense our self-imposed limitations and some of the blind spots in our thinking.

Reflection is about quieting down your mind so that answers can arise within the quietness. Often, when we're looking for an answer, we "turn up the volume" of our thinking. We think, think, think—and then we think some more.

People who regularly use reflection, on the other hand, understand that we are a part of a deeper intelligence. The only factor preventing us from hearing or being connected to this wisdom is the chatter of our own thinking. When we turn down the volume of our thinking, we can begin to sense this deeper intelligence. This is reflection.

58.

DON'T ALLOW PASSING THOUGHTS TO TURN INTO ISSUES

Thousands of thoughts pass through our minds each and every day. These thoughts are made up of our ideas, plans, expectations, and memories, among other things. Some of our thoughts are happy; many are not.

As thoughts pass through the mind, essentially one of two things can happen. First, my thought can be a passing thought. Most of our thoughts fall into this category. The other possibility is that I hold that thought in my mind, as if to examine it. I keep it right there, "in my face," where I can study it. I give it my undivided attention and attach significance to it.

You can probably sense how easy it can be to create an issue over practically anything. All that's really required is that you continue feeding the thought with your attention. The problem is, if you don't see how your own thinking contributes to the issues that frustrate you, you will always blame others.

The solution is to be willing to accept the fact that many annoyances are simply passing thoughts that we are taking a little too seriously. The next time you find yourself feeling irritated, check in with your thinking. See whether you might be holding on to something instead of simply dropping it or letting it pass by.

59.

DON'T SWEAT THE BUREAUCRACY

I can't imagine that there are very many people who work for a living who don't have to deal with at least some form of bureaucracy. You can, of course, spend your entire lifetime complaining about bureaucracy, wishing it would disappear, and fighting every step of the way. In the end, however, you're still going to have to deal with it. My suggestion is to stop sweating it and, in fact, strive to make peace with bureaucracy. This can be done.

Let me make myself perfectly clear. I'm not suggesting that you roll over and become a victim of bureaucracy. What I am suggesting is that you find a way to maximize your efficiency when you must deal with bureaucracy, do the very best that you can with it, make suggestions on ways to improve the system, and then detach yourself from the craziness. And you know what else? Most people who work for a bureaucracy are just as frustrated as you and I. For the most part, they are really nice people who are, to some degree, trapped in a role.

So the lesson is this: The more you are able to keep your bearings and composure, and have some perspective, the more likely it is that you will find one of these nice people to help you.

60.

LAUGH AT YOUR MISTAKES (AND YOU WON'T REPEAT THEM)

Have you ever noticed that the more seriously you take your mistakes, the more you make them? And the more seriously you take your problems, the more you create them? This is because your behavior follows your attention. When your mind is full of mistakes and problems, your attention is riveted in a negative direction. Thus, when you make a big deal out of something you have done wrong, when you take yourself too seriously, you are actually setting the stage to repeat the mistake.

However, energy cuts both ways. If your energy is abundant, your mind will be in a more creative mode—searching for solutions and building on strengths. Your mind will be open to suggestions to new and better ways of doing things. It is far more powerful to be in favor of something positive than to be against something negative—*for* peace instead of against violence, *for* excellence instead of against mediocrity.

A decision to remain lighthearted doesn't mean you don't care. It simply means that you refuse to compound a problem by making a bigger deal out of something than is appropriate. It means that you understand the value of keeping your perspective and sense of humor, even in the face of adversity. In every mistake there is the potential for growth.

61.

ASK YOURSELF, "WILL THIS MATTER A YEAR FROM NOW?"

Almost every day I play a game with myself that I call "time warp." I made it up in response to my consistent, erroneous belief that what I was all worked up about was really important.

To play time warp, all you have to do is imagine that whatever circumstance you are dealing with isn't happening right now but a year from now. Then simply ask yourself, "Is this situation really as important as I'm making it out to be?" Once in a great while it may be—but most of the time, it simply isn't.

Whether it be an argument with your spouse, child, or boss, a mistake, a lost opportunity, a lost wallet, a work-related rejection, or a sprained ankle, chances are that a year from now you aren't going to care. It will be one more irrelevant detail in your life. While this simple game won't solve all your problems, it can give you an enormous amount of needed perspective. I find myself laughing at things that I used to take far too seriously. Now, rather than using up my energy feeling angry and overwhelmed, I can use it instead on spending time with my wife and children or engaging in creative thinking.

62.

MAKE THE FRESH-START COMMITMENT

Making the fresh-start commitment means making the decision to drop all concerns, regrets, and disappointments from your past, as well as all of your expectations regarding the future. Today becomes the focal point of your life. This day becomes more important than past mistakes or future plans. You stop comparing today to days gone by—or your hopes of a better tomorrow. You ask yourself the question, "How can I make today the best day that it can possibly be?" The answer to this simple question becomes the key to a heartfelt and loving connection.

It's been said that "yesterday is but a dream, tomorrow a fantasy." Today, however, is reality—the only day that is guaranteed to be yours. The good news is that you have the capacity to make the precious moments of today all that they can be. You do so by dismissing your thoughts from the past and postponing your reactions of tomorrow—until they, too, become today. The trick is to forgive your past, become less fearful of the future, and bless the gift of today.

The nice thing about this strategy is that it's easy and it really works. The present moments of your life are special and powerful. By immersing yourself in them, you give yourself the capacity to make every day the best day of your life.

63.

REMEMBER THE PHRASE, "BEING DEAD IS BAD FOR BUSINESS"

I'll bet you can guess where I'm going with this one. You can, of course, easily extend this clever phrase to the way we treat ourselves—particularly in the areas of our personal health. The saying holds true however you look at it. Being dead is bad for business.

This line really helps to keep things in perspective when we get overloaded with work. For example, when you find yourself saying things like, "I don't have time to exercise," what you really should be saying is, "I don't have time not to exercise." If you lose your health and sense of well-being, you won't make it to work at all. In the long run, it takes far less time to take care of yourself than it does to lose your ability to function well.

By remembering that "being dead is bad for business," you'll probably begin taking better care of yourself—physically and emotionally. You'll feel better, be happier, and probably live longer. You can let go of your fear that you'll fall behind because, in fact, you'll be more productive and have a longer, happier career. So keep yourself alive and healthy. It's good for business.

64.

SURRENDER TO THE FACT THAT LIFE ISN'T FAIR

A friend of mine asked me the question, "Who said life was going to be fair, or that it was even meant to be fair?" Her question was a good one. It reminded me of something I was taught as a youngster: Life isn't fair. It's a bummer, but it's absolutely true. Ironically, recognizing this sobering fact can be a very liberating insight.

One of the nice things about surrendering to the fact that life isn't fair is that it keeps us from feeling sorry for ourselves by encouraging us to do the very best we can with what we have. We know it's not "life's job" to make everything perfect; it's our own challenge.

The fact that life isn't fair doesn't mean we shouldn't do everything in our power to improve our own lives or the world as a whole. To the contrary, it suggests that we should. When we don't recognize or admit that life isn't fair, we tend to feel pity for others and for ourselves. Pity is a self-defeating emotion that does nothing for anyone. When we do recognize that life isn't fair, however, we feel compassion for others and for ourselves. And compassion is a heartfelt emotion that delivers loving-kindness to everyone it touches.

65.

ASK FOR WHAT YOU WANT

Jack Canfield and Mark Victor Hansen, authors of *Chicken Soup for the Soul*, call this simple strategy the "Aladdin Factor." It's astonishing what you can accomplish by simply asking for what you want—help, a raise, forgiveness, another chance, or something else.

If it's so obviously helpful to ask for what we want, why do so few of us do it? Once again, the answer is fear. We worry about the outcome. We're afraid of rejection or a negative response. We might be worried about offending someone or being perceived as weak, or of taking advantage of our relationship.

Several years ago, I had the realization that one of my own greatest assets was *my* willingness to help others. Hundreds of times, I've returned calls to complete strangers. With friends and family, my willingness to help is even greater. I realized that feeling needed and wanted is a deep and important human need.

Despite our fears, it's actually quite arrogant and self-righteous to assume that others aren't as willing to help. The key in asking for something is to be sincere in your belief that, deep down, others *want* to help you. Approach your request by assuming that the person you are asking is just like you—they have an inner longing to be of help.

66.

ALLOW YOURSELF TO BE BORED

I was first exposed to the idea that occasional boredom can be beneficial while studying with a therapist in a tiny little town in Washington. After finishing our first day together, I asked my instructor, "What is there to do around here at night?" He responded by saying, "What I'd like you to do is allow yourself to be bored. Do nothing. This is part of your training." He went on to explain that if you allow yourself to be bored, even for an hour—or less—and don't fight it, the feelings of boredom will be replaced with feelings of peace and relaxation.

Much to my surprise, he was absolutely right. At first, I could barely stand it. I was so used to doing something every second that I struggled to relax. But after a while I got used to it, and have long since learned to enjoy just "being," rather than "doing," for a few minutes each day.

Much of our anxiety and inner struggle stems from our busy, overactive minds always needing something to entertain them, something to focus on, and always wondering, "What's next?"

The beauty of doing nothing is that it teaches you to clear your mind and relax. It allows your mind the freedom to "not know," for a brief period of time.

67.

TAKE RESPONSIBILITY FOR YOUR OWN HAPPINESS

It's a little scary to listen to many of the most popular songs on the radio. So often the message is, "You make me happy; I'd be lost without you; you are my world," or other messages that take away all the power and responsibility to make yourself happy and put it on someone else. That's an enormous amount of pressure to put on another person.

On the surface, this concept seems rather obvious, but how many of us really do take full responsibility for our own happiness?

If you believe that the answer to your unhappiness lies in someone else's hands (no matter how much you love them), you're in for a load of trouble. Don't get us wrong. We're not saying other people don't play a role in your happiness. However, ultimately, you and you alone are responsible for making yourself happy. When your life isn't working, you may have to make difficult choices, have painful or uncomfortable discussions, or compromise in some way—but you have to take responsibility for your own level of happiness.

This is a very empowering insight. You'll be amazed at how much happier you'll be when you put the responsibility for your own happiness where it belongs—with you.

68.

DON'T PANIC!

In business, people panic about practically everything—missed deadlines, orders not received, comments by others, fear of mistakes, negative trends. You name it and someone has panicked about it. Yet I've never seen even a single instance where the panic actually helped to solve the problem. Instead, panic is neutral at best and greatly interferes at worst. Panic tends to bring out the worst in everyone. It makes others (and you) feel tense and fearful. It increases the likelihood of mistakes, missed opportunities, and miscommunication.

When you make the commitment to stop panicking, you'll notice some incredible things happening. First, you'll notice that a vast majority of what you are most worried about will never happen, or it won't be as bad as you feared. Benjamin Franklin said, "Some terrible things happened in my lifetime—a few of which actually happened." Second, when you learn to keep your bearings, your wisdom will come forth. In the absence of worry, answers will emerge. Finally, when you stay calm, you really do bring out the best in others. If you can maintain your bearings, chances are the people around you will, too.

Life is far too short to worry it away.

69.

LIGHT A CANDLE INSTEAD OF CURSING THE DARKNESS

As the title suggests, this strategy involves taking positive, solution-oriented steps (however small) toward improving a situation instead of complaining about what's wrong. It means being more a part of the solution rather than a reminder or reinforcement of the problem. I've found that work is the ideal environment to practice this philosophy.

In many instances, you can not only make a dent in a problem but actually reduce your own stress level in the process by simply choosing to "light a candle." Simply put, this means making a suggestion or taking a positive step toward improving a source of stress. It means putting increased emphasis on a potential solution and less emphasis on "cursing" the problem.

For example, suppose gossip or talking behind others' backs is a problem where you work. Rather than remaining resentful, see if you can make a tiny dent in the problem. Gather together a few of your friends and gently bring the issue to the table. Instead of accusing anyone, focus on your own contribution. Confess that you have been as guilty as anyone else in indulging in occasional gossip, and state that you're going to make a genuine effort not to do so. Invite others to join you.

See how easy it is to light a candle?

70.

BANISH YOUR DOUBT

In your dreams you can do some remarkable things—be two places at once, shift scenes and environments, walk through walls, become rich and famous, overcome great obstacles, get along with your parents, to name just a few. And through it all, you never, ever doubt your abilities.

Yet in our waking state, most of us spend a great deal of energy, every day of our lives, doubting our abilities—to our great detriment. We doubt ourselves at practically every turn.

For years I convinced myself that I couldn't speak in front of groups. I believed this self-imposed limitation with all my heart. Then one day a friend and mentor put me on the spot in front of a large group. Before it was my turn to speak, he turned to me and said, "Richard, the idea that you aren't capable of speaking to a group is absolutely preposterous. Dismiss this crazy notion from your mind and everything will be fine. Get over it, now!" I remember his words as if they were said this morning. He was right. Speaking became effortless the *moment* I banished the doubt from my mind.

You can do the same thing. Whatever doubts are lingering in your mind, let them go. It's far easier than you think, and it will produce great rewards.

71.

LOWER YOUR TOLERANCE TO STRESS

In my work as a stress consultant, I hear the proud words "I have a very high tolerance to stress" almost daily. When these stressed-out people first arrive at my office, they are often hoping for strategies to raise their tolerance to stress even higher so they can handle even more!

Fortunately, there is an inviolable law in our emotional environment that goes something like this: Our current level of stress will be exactly that of our tolerance to stress. If you teach people to raise their tolerance to stress, they will accept even more confusion and responsibility until their external level of stress matches that of their tolerance.

Instead, start noticing your stress early, before it gets out of hand. When you feel your mind moving too quickly, it's time to back off and regain your bearings. When you're feeling out of control and resentful of all you have to do, a better strategy is to relax, take a few deep breaths, and go for a short walk.

When your mind is clear and peaceful and your stress level is reduced, you'll be more effective and you'll have more fun. As you lower your tolerance to stress, you will find that you'll have far less stress to handle, as well as creative ideas for handling the stress that is left over.

72.

STOP BEING SO DEFENSIVE

If you could eliminate all defensiveness in your personality, you would not only have the best relationships in town but, in fact, you would become the most loving and adorable person on this planet. You'd have so much charisma and charm, you'd be almost irresistible, a virtual magnet for human companionship.

Let's be realistic. No one can eliminate all their defensive reactions; it's part of being human. However, with some gentle effort, it's relatively easy to make great strides in the direction of becoming less defensive.

The alternative to feeling or acting defensive is called acceptance. Unlike defensiveness, which is like tightening your fist and becoming stubborn, acceptance is like releasing your fist and becoming open and receptive. When you strive for acceptance, you are attempting to receive life—including criticism, comments you disagree with, and all the rest—with a degree of equanimity.

Acceptance is not about becoming a doormat, nor is it about changing your most treasured beliefs. Instead, acceptance is about becoming slightly more open and receptive to what others have to say. It's about becoming less reactive and a better listener.

Why not give it a try? What have you got to lose, other than a habitual response that interferes with your relationships being all that they can be?

73.

CREATE FROM THE INSIDE OUT

You can work long and hard, be creative, clever, talented, insightful, even lucky—but if you fail to understand the importance of your own thoughts in the process of creation, it will all be for naught.

The single most important factor of building a life you love comes from within yourself—your thoughts. As James Allen reminds us in *As a Man Thinketh*, "A particular train of thought persisted in, be it good or bad, cannot fail to produce its results on the character and circumstances. A man cannot directly choose his circumstances, but he can choose his thoughts, and so indirectly, yet surely, shape his circumstances."

I've known many successful people in many different fields. Although they have vastly different talents, temperaments, skills, work ethics, and backgrounds, they all have one thing in common. This golden thread of consistency is that each of them sees him- or herself as successful. They never question this fact; they can't understand why anyone would question their own level of greatness. Success originates in the mind and translates into the material world. It doesn't work the other way around, as so many seem to believe. Successful people know that the one aspect of life that they do have control over is their own thinking. All of us have this same advantage, so let's all start there!

74.

ONCE A WEEK, WRITE A HEARTFELT LETTER

This is an exercise that has helped to change many lives, assisting people in becoming more peaceful and loving. Taking a few minutes each week to write a heartfelt letter does many things for you. Picking up a pen or typing on a keyboard slows you down long enough to remember the beautiful people in your life. The act of sitting down to write helps to fill your life with gratitude.

You'll probably be amazed at how many people appear on your letter list. I had one client who said, "I probably don't have enough weeks left in my life to write everyone on my list." This may or may not be true for you, but chances are, there are many people in your life, or from your past, who are quite deserving of a friendly, heartfelt letter. Even if you don't have people in your life to whom you feel you can write, go ahead and write the letter to someone you don't know instead—perhaps to an author who may not even be living, whose works you admire. Part of the value of the letter is to gear your thinking toward gratitude. Writing the letter, even if it isn't sent, would do just that.

Write your first letter this week. I'll bet you'll be glad you did.

75.

KNOW THE SECRET OF SILENCE

Have you ever noticed that when you are quiet and still, calm and silent, you know exactly what to do? Being silent doesn't shut down your mind, it only activates a deeper type of intelligence. No one knows for sure where this deeper intelligence comes from, or what it's called, but all wise cultures are certain that it exists.

Learning to trust in silence is simple because, when you do, the results are so spectacular. Once you get the hang of it your life will become far easier and less stressful. The next time you need an answer that is not readily available, rather than racking your brain over it, try an experiment. Instead of actively thinking about the issue, let it go. The fact that you know the nature of the problem or question is all the information you need. Allow the question to settle, like silt in water.

Like the back burner of a stove, the question or problem begins to bubble. In time—it may be a few minutes, hours, or days, depending on the issue—an answer will pop into your head. You may be surprised, but you'll certainly be delighted at the wisdom that comes through. Be careful, however, not to take yourself too seriously. The wisdom you experience comes not from you but from the silence.

76.

BE CONSISTENTLY GRATEFUL

Gratitude is important for many reasons. It keeps your heart open and your mind receptive to the gifts of life. It serves as a constant reminder of how fortunate you are to be alive, and keeps you from taking your relationships for granted. Gratitude keeps you feeling satisfied, reminding you that what you have is good enough. When you are focused on gratitude, it keeps your problems in perspective, especially the small ones. It immunizes you from being bothered by your partner's little quirks or the imperfections in your work. Gratitude allows you to see beyond the "small stuff" and keeps you from overreacting to the hassles you encounter.

Beyond your own satisfaction, however, the expression of gratitude strengthens your relationships. Everyone loves to know (and hear) that they are appreciated and valued. In fact, when someone feels taken for granted, or underappreciated, resentment or apathy is usually not too far away.

With some gentle attention, it's also easy to develop an "attitude of gratitude." You start by taking your focus off of what's wrong and what's not working, and replacing that focus with a sincere commitment to reflect on all that's right in your life. That's it! The rest will take care of itself.

77.

JOIN MY NEW CLUB, "TGIT"

Until now, the world was primarily made of two clubs. The most popular club, by far, was the "TGIF" club, or "Thank God It's Friday." To be a member of this club, your primary focus is on the weekend. Most members are highly stressed because only two days of the week are considered "good days."

The other business club is substantially smaller, yet in some ways the members are more dedicated to the club. This one is called "TGIM," or "Thank God It's Monday." These members are usually workaholics who can't stand weekends because they are away from work!

I invite you to join an alternate club. This new club is called "TGIT," or "Thank God It's Today." Members of this club are happy seven days a week because they understand that every day is unique, and each brings with it different gifts. Members of this club are grateful to be alive; they rejoice in their many blessings and expect each day to be full of wonder, surprise, and opportunity.

Just think: If you wake up every day of the week with an attitude of "I'm glad today is today. I'm going to make this day as positive and wonderful as I possibly can," you may be surprised at how much less stressed you'll be.

78.

IMAGINE YOURSELF AT YOUR OWN FUNERAL

This strategy is a little scary for some people but universally effective at reminding us of what's most important in our lives.

When we look back on our lives, how many of us are going to be pleased at how uptight we were? Almost universally, when people look back on their lives while on their deathbed, they wish that their priorities had been quite different. With few exceptions, people wish they hadn't "sweated the small stuff" so much. Instead, they wish they had spent more time with the people and activities that they truly loved and less time worrying about aspects of life that, upon deeper examination, really don't matter all that much. Imagining yourself at your own funeral allows you to look back at your life while you still have the chance to make some important changes.

While it can be a little scary or painful, it's a good idea to consider your own death and, in the process, your life. Doing so will remind you of the kind of person you want to be and the priorities that are most important to you. If you're at all like me, you'll probably get a wake-up call that can be an excellent source of change.

79.

NEVER UNDERESTIMATE THE VALUE OF GOODWILL

I once had a signed contract to do a speaking engagement. Because I had agreed to do the event, I had to turn down several far more lucrative offers. Then, very close to the date of the engagement, the company canceled the event and asked if I'd be willing to switch times.

Clearly, I had the ethical and legal right to decline their request and collect my fee. But I didn't. Instead, I agreed to switch dates and did so without complaining. They were so thrilled and grateful. And my decision has paid handsome dividends. I've received numerous offers since that time that I believe are linked to my willingness to be flexible.

So, what is goodwill—having others think highly of you—really worth? I don't think there's any way to quantify it, but it's certainly valuable. The problem is, it doesn't always work so smoothly. Our goodwill efforts are not always appreciated. Some people take advantage of others, and you never know if or when your goodwill efforts will pay off. Yet if you have faith that being fair and ethical and going the extra mile is the right thing to do, then, over time, you will be rewarded.

80.

REPEAT TO YOURSELF, "LIFE ISN'T AN EMERGENCY"

In some ways, this strategy epitomizes the essential message of this book. The truth is, life isn't an emergency.

I've had hundreds of clients over the years who have all but neglected their families as well as their own dreams because of their propensity to believe that life is an emergency. They justify their neurotic behavior by believing that if they don't work eighty hours a week, they won't get everything done.

A client who is a homemaker and mother of three children recently said to me, "I just can't get the house cleaned up the way I like it before everyone leaves in the morning." She was acting (and feeling) like there was a gun pointed at her head and the sniper was demanding that every dish be put away—or else! The silent assumption was *This is an emergency!* The truth was, no one other than her had created the pressure she was experiencing.

I've never met anyone (myself included) who hasn't turned little things into great big emergencies. We take our own goals so seriously that we forget to have fun along the way. We take simple preferences and turn them into conditions for our own happiness. Practice having the humility to admit that, in most cases, you're creating your own emergencies.

81.

DELIGHT IN THE SUCCESS OF OTHERS

Let's be honest here. Have you ever found yourself secretly wishing someone else would fail? I don't mean you wish them any serious bad luck, only that they don't become even more successful than you? Sometimes it's hard to wish others well, particularly those you know well—friends, colleagues, neighbors, family members. We're human; we get jealous.

And yet the way to rise to the top is to wish everyone well, to hope with all your heart that everyone can expand to their greatest potential, to wish that the people you know, and those whom you don't know, can all realize their dreams and achieve greatness.

As people achieve their goals, the pie gets even bigger for everyone. We don't want to see one another at our lowest common denominator, but at our highest common vision. We can *all* succeed and each time someone does—anyone—it helps the rest of us. When you delight in the success of others, it's as if you are sprinkling the seeds for a garden of success.

As you wish others well, notice how good it feels. When your wishes are sincere, they will serve as a reminder that giving and receiving are two sides of the same coin. Truly, it feels as good to see someone else succeed as it does to succeed yourself.

82.

DON'T SWEAT THE DEMANDING BOSS

I'd estimate that a large percentage of adults that I know are either working for, or have worked for, a demanding boss.

We can, like most do, complain about them, wish they would go away, and feel forever stressed about the situation. Or we can try (hard as it is) to stay focused on the positive aspects of the demanding party.

One "saving grace" I realized about demanding people is that, generally speaking, they are demanding to everyone. In other words, it's not personal.

Years ago, I was having a difficult time working with a demanding editor, when a friend asked me a very important question. She said, "Has it ever occurred to you that the most demanding people are often the ones who push you out of your comfort zone and help you rise to a new level of competence?" Until that moment, it hadn't occurred to me that this was true.

The realization that there are two sides to demanding people—positive and negative—has made my entire life, especially my work life, a whole lot easier. Whereas before I would become defensive and dread the process, I now approach demanding people in an entirely new way. I'm open to what they may have to teach me, and I don't take their behavior personally.

83.

ASK YOURSELF THE QUESTION, "IN THE SCHEME OF THINGS, IS THIS REALLY THAT BIG A DEAL?"

When you get right down to it, at the heart of learning not to sweat the small stuff is the art of beginning to recognize that many of the things that we treat as a really big deal...aren't. We blow things out of proportion; we read into things, anticipate the worst, get uptight, rehearse unhappiness in our mind, and turn molehills into mountains. Once we turn the corner, however, and begin to put things into their proper perspective, we're on the road to a more peaceful life.

Simple as it sounds (and it is simple), it can be enormously helpful to ask yourself the question, "In the scheme of things, is this really that big a deal?" In most cases, the simple act of asking the question is all that needs to be done. The question will gently but firmly jolt you into reality, and immediately you'll become more reflective and increase your level of perspective.

A friend once told me, "If someone is dying, seriously hurt, or in serious danger, it's a really big deal. Otherwise, it's really not." I certainly haven't mastered this strategy, but I know I'm moving in the right direction. And you can, too!

84.

REMEMBER THE GOLDEN RULE

Do you remember the golden rule? It goes like this: "Do unto others as you would have them do unto you." What are some other ways of saying this magical formula? "What goes around, comes around." "As you treat others, so shall you be treated." "If you don't have something nice to say, don't say anything at all." There are many variations, and it's one of the first lessons we try to teach our children.

Simply put, all you have to do to ensure that you will be treated fairly, respectfully, and with kindness—and to ensure that others will reach out to help you and praise you—is to do these things yourself!

Become a thoughtful person. Offer assistance. Be nice. Reach out to others. Become even more generous. Say "Thank you." These, and hundreds of other similar little gestures, are the ways you can reach out and tell the world you care.

Don't make the mistake of becoming upset or frustrated if your acts of kindness don't come back immediately. The universe has its own set of rules and its own sense of timing. Be patient and loving. If you are committed to the golden rule, it's only a matter of time before your life will be filled with everything you desire.

85.

EXPERIMENT WITH YOUR BACK BURNER

Your back burner is an excellent tool for remembering a fact or bringing forth an insight. It's an almost effortless yet effective way of using your mind when you might otherwise start feeling stressed out. Using your back burner means allowing your mind to solve a problem while you are busy doing something else, here in the present moment.

The back burner of your mind works in the same way as the back burner of a stove. While on low heat, the cooking process mixes, blends, and simmers the ingredients into a tasty meal. The way you prepared this meal was to throw the various ingredients into the pot, mix them up, and leave them alone. Often, the less you interfere, the better the result.

In much the same way, we can solve many of life's problems (serious and otherwise) if we feed the back burner of our mind with a list of problems, facts, and variables, and possible solutions.

Whether you are struggling to solve a problem or can't remember a person's name, your back burner puts your quieter, softer, and sometimes most intelligent source of thinking to work. Gently hold the problem in your mind without actively analyzing it. This simple technique will help you solve many problems and will greatly reduce the stress and effort in your life.

86.

DON'T CONTINUE DOING THE SAME THING AND EXPECT DIFFERENT RESULTS

My family was visiting an aquarium when we observed a most curious thing. For about fifteen minutes we watched a beautiful sea turtle swim gracefully around a large tank. Each time the turtle would pass, he would bump his fin and part of his head into the glass, in exactly the same way. It was clear that he wasn't being hurt, but it did appear to the untrained eye that each time he hit the glass, he was quite surprised.

How often do we overreact, sweat the small stuff, or respond in a knee-jerk manner to someone we love (our partner or potential partner, our child, a colleague, a parent), and receive, in return, a response we don't like? Then, the next time we're frustrated, we use the same response with the same result. You'd think after thousands and thousands of attempts, we'd get the message. But usually we don't!

Whether it's our typical reaction to criticism or suggestions or something totally different—there is usually some way that we do the same thing over and over yet expect a different response. By making an honest assessment of your own tendencies, you can nip this problem in the bud. In doing so, your relationships will improve, and you'll save yourself a great deal of frustration.

87.

STAY AWAY FROM THE BLAME GAME

One of the most insidious, tempting habits in all of life also happens to be one of the surest ways to rob yourself of empowerment, joy, and abundance. I'm referring to the habit of blaming others or external conditions for our failures, mistakes, problems, and lack of success.

Blaming others is a very easy thing to do. We might attribute our lack of fulfillment to changing times, a missed opportunity, or too little education. Or, we might complain to our wife or husband, "I travel too much to consider that new opportunity." How about this one: "I'd be in better shape, it's just that I don't have time."

It's not that our tendency to blame is without any merit. There usually is a grain of truth in our complaints. But all that does is keep the game going. It's really easy to blame our lack of exercise or family involvement on our schedule—it's a little tougher to admit that we are not prioritizing it.

If you can have the humility to admit that you, too, fall into this habit from time to time—and you can identify those instances—you will have opened the door and paved the way for almost unlimited success and enjoyment in whatever it is that you do.

88.

SPEND A MOMENT EVERY DAY THINKING OF SOMEONE TO THANK

This simple strategy, which may take only a few seconds to complete, has long been one of the most important habits I have ever engaged in. I try to remember to start my day thinking of someone to thank. To me, gratitude and inner peace go hand in hand. Gratitude, then, is worthy of a little practice.

If you're anything like me, you probably have many people in your life to feel grateful for: friends, family members, people from your past, teachers, gurus, people from work, someone who gave you a break, as well as countless others. You may want to thank a higher power for the gift of life itself, or for the beauty of nature.

As you think of people to be grateful for, remember that it can be anyone—someone who allowed you to merge into traffic, someone who held the door open for you, or a physician who saved your life. The point is to gear your attention toward gratitude, preferably first thing in the morning.

It may seem like an awfully simple suggestion, but it really works! If you wake up in the morning with gratitude on your mind, it's pretty difficult, in fact almost impossible, to feel anything but peace.

89.

LET GO OF THE FEAR THAT IF YOU'RE RELAXED OR HAPPY, YOU'RE GOING TO FAIL

Sadly, many people believe that if you aren't uptight and serious, you are doomed to failure. In my entire lifetime, I've never been more convinced that something is not true. Let me give you an analogy:

Think back to last year's Thanksgiving dinner. Remember how you felt after eating all that food. You likely felt stuffed and tired. When you eat too much, the energy that is usually directed toward normal body functions—healing, cell division, metabolism, and all sorts of other good stuff—must go toward digestion. This makes you feel sleepy and lethargic. You lose motivation and energy.

You can extend this same metaphor to your tendency to be overly serious and immobilized over little things. When you are angry, bothered, and annoyed, virtually all the mental and emotional energy that could otherwise be used for creativity, spontaneity, and mental ambition is taken away. When you focus on things that irritate you, it interferes with the process of creation.

As you lighten up, relax, and unwind, you open the doors of creativity and joy that were previously hidden. You discover new interests and new possibilities. So, starting today, remind yourself that it's okay to relax—in fact, it's more than okay, it's downright important.

90.

MAKE PEACE WITH CHANGE

It's been said that there are only two certainties in life—death and taxes. Not true. A third certainty, one that is constant and must be dealt with on a day-to-day, moment-to-moment basis, is change. And one of the greatest gifts you can give yourself is to be at peace with this fact of life.

Although we often wish it were otherwise, nothing stays the same. Our bodies change, as does our health. We can fight it, but change continues. Our moods change, almost constantly, as do our perceptions. One moment we feel inspired and loving—then, out of the blue, we experience doubt or fear. A few hours later, we're back on track.

When you resist change, you're never more than a moment away from disappointment. Whether you know it or not, you're always on guard because you're either trying to keep things the same if you like what you're experiencing—or you're fighting to make things different.

Embracing change means that you stop demanding that life be other than it really is in this moment. When you embrace rather than resist change, you begin to accept and usually enjoy each moment as it arises.

There is tremendous freedom that comes with the acceptance of change.

91.

SMILE AT STRANGERS, LOOK INTO THEIR EYES, AND SAY HELLO

Have you ever noticed or thought about how little eye contact most of us have with strangers? Why? Are we afraid of them? What keeps us from opening our hearts to people we don't know?

There is virtually always a parallel between our attitude toward strangers and our overall level of happiness. In other words, it's unusual to find a person who walks around with her head down, frowning and looking away from people, who is secretly a peaceful, joyful person.

I'm not suggesting it's better to be outgoing than introverted, that you need to expend tons of extra energy trying to brighten others' days, or that you should pretend to be friendly. I am suggesting, however, that if you think of strangers as being a little more like you and treat them not only with kindness and respect but with smiles and eye contact as well, you'll probably notice some pretty nice changes in yourself. You'll begin to see that most people are just like you. When you see how similar we all are, you begin to see the innocence in all of us. Along with seeing the innocence in people comes a profound feeling of inner happiness.

92.

WHISTLE WHILE YOU WORK

It's amazing what happens when you act as if you love what you do. The positive energy helps not only you but everyone around you. It's contagious.

One of my favorite "Peanuts" cartoon strips was one where Charlie Brown was hanging his head low. He was depressed. While his head was down and his shoulders were slumped over, he was explaining to Linus that if you want to be depressed, it's really important to look depressed. He went on to correctly explain that if you were to lift your head up and smile, it would take you out of your depression and make you feel better!

The idea of whistling while you work is identical, only it's on the opposite end of the attitudinal spectrum. When you appreciate the privilege of doing whatever you are doing, it makes it virtually impossible to feel down. Instead of complaining, you'll notice all the things you love about your work and your life. It will keep your thinking fresh and spontaneous, alive and interesting. The people around you will be affected, too. They will actually listen to what you have to say, and they will appreciate you more than ever before.

Starting today, see if you can incorporate a "whistle while you work" attitude into your daily routine.

93.

DON'T GET STRESSED BY THE PREDICTABLE

In many industries there are certain standard procedures or problems that are, to a large degree, predictable. The first few times they happen, or if you're caught off guard, it's understandable that they can create some anxiety or stress. However, once you factor them into your awareness, and you can predict how events are typically played out, it's silly to be annoyed and upset.

I met a police officer who took it personally when people would drive faster than the speed limit. He would get frustrated and dish out harsh lectures, apparently forgetting that it was his job to catch people speeding to create safer roads. This is a predictable part of his work.

Before you say, "I'd never get upset over something like that," take a careful look at your own industry. It's always easier to see why someone else shouldn't be upset than it is to admit that you, too, can make a bigger deal out of something than is really necessary.

As you see these and other work-related tendencies in their proper "predictable" perspective, you can eliminate a great deal of stress. You can make allowances in your mind, attitude, and behavior for that which you know is going to happen anyway. You can breathe easier and, perhaps, learn to relax a little more.

94.

REMEMBER TO ACKNOWLEDGE

I can't think of a single person who doesn't love and appreciate being acknowledged. On the flip side, most people either resent, or at least feel slighted by not being acknowledged. This being the case, this one seems like a "no-brainer."

You can acknowledge others in many ways. When someone calls you, acknowledge the call. When they send you something, remember to say thank you, or take the time to write a note. When someone does a good job, say so. When they apologize, acknowledge that, too. It's especially important to acknowledge acts of kindness—doing so reinforces the act and encourages more of the same. We all benefit.

We should acknowledge others, not simply to get something in return, but because it's the right thing to do—because it makes them feel good. People remember acknowledgment and they appreciate it. When you need a favor or advice, the fact that you have previously taken the time to acknowledge someone often comes back to help you.

So think about it. Does someone in your life deserve some sort of acknowledgment? If so, what's holding you up?

95.

RESPOND WITH LOVE

When you respond with love—not jealousy, anger, resentment, selfishness, or frustration, but simply love—you've all but guaranteed a loving interaction and, in the long run, a loving and successful partnership. Rather than sweating the small stuff, you'll be appreciating the big stuff! You'll be nondefensive, nonreactive, and accepting. You'll find that everything important in your relationships will magically fall into place, including the difficulties. The reason: love heals. When you respond with love, those you love respect you, love you, want to be with you, and want you to be happy. Compromise is easy, as is forgiveness.

I've thought a great deal about this idea, and I simply can't poke any holes in it. Every great spiritual teacher and respected spiritual tradition advocates this position—and every great spiritual book is filled with this wisdom. Further, when you talk to happy couples about their suggestions for a strong relationship, this is always, 100 percent of the time, at or near the top of their list.

It's been said and expressed in so many different ways, but the message is the same—simply put, "Respond with love, and all will be well."

96.

DON'T SWEAT THE SETBACKS

The question isn't *if* we will have setbacks, disappointments, and failures in business (and in life)—we will. Rather, the question is how we will deal with them. Will we, as so many do, sweat it? Will we become upset, immobilized, or pessimistic? Or will we take a more positive approach?

In hindsight, it's usually easy to see that most setbacks are nothing more than "small stuff" disguised as big stuff. They can seem significant, even insurmountable in the moment. Yet once we get through them, we look back on setbacks and even failures as a necessary, even important part of our success.

I once heard a speaker use the example of people driving around, looking for a parking place. He said, "It's as if people are driving around looking for no place to park." What he meant was that many people get frustrated because most of the spaces are full. It's easy to forget that you don't need a bunch of spaces—you only need one; the others are irrelevant. Simple as this seems, it's actually an important point to remember—you don't need everything to go perfectly, you only need a few things to go right. And once they do, the setbacks simply fade away. Remembering this takes a great deal of pressure and frustration off your shoulders.

97.

SET ASIDE QUIET TIME, EVERY DAY

As I begin to write this strategy, it's exactly 4:30 in the morning, my favorite time of the day. I still have at least an hour and a half before my wife and children get out of bed and the phone begins to ring. It's absolutely silent outside, and I'm in complete solitude. There is something rejuvenating and peaceful about being alone and having some time to reflect, work, or simply enjoy the quiet.

Whether it's ten minutes of meditation or yoga, spending a little time in nature, or locking the bathroom door and taking a ten-minute bath, quiet time to yourself is a vital part of life. Like spending time alone, it helps to balance the noise and confusion that infiltrate much of our day.

There's a little ritual that I do that I've shared with many friends. Like many people, I drive to and from my office. On my way home from work, as I get close to my driveway, I pull my car over and stop. There is a nice spot where I can spend a minute or two looking at the view or closing my eyes and breathing. It slows me down and helps me feel centered and grateful. With a simple shift in my actions, I enter my home feeling much more relaxed.

98.

BUILD UP A LARGE "TRUST FUND"

I grew up believing that only very wealthy (usually spoiled) people had the privilege of a "trust fund." Not true! Each individual has the kind of trust fund that really matters: the trust of other people. The only question is: How large is it?

The way to build a large trust fund is simple and straightforward. It involves being accountable for your actions, however large or small, doing what you say you are going to do, delivering on your promises, and so forth. Accountability is derived in both small and large doses. For example, if you tell someone you are going to call them at three o'clock, or pick them up at the airport, and you do so, you earn small credits toward your trust fund. If you don't do what you say you're going to do, while any individual action or inaction may not seem like a very big deal, it reduces the size of your trust fund.

Obviously, no one is perfect. But starting today, behave with your trust fund in mind. Before you say you are going to do something that someone else is going to depend on, check in with yourself. Ask yourself, "Will I be able to keep this commitment?" Remember, the size of your trust fund depends on it.

99.

LOOK IN THE MIRROR

So often, when we're angry or frustrated at the one we love, something else is secretly going on beneath the surface—we're angry or frustrated at ourselves. That's right, ourselves. But because it's easier to put the blame on someone else, we often blame others instead of looking in the mirror.

Shortly after we had our first child, Kris and I went through a brief period of time when I was unusually frustrated at what I thought was her. I expressed frustration that I was "doing too much"—working full time, attending graduate school, and trying to be a good father.

Kris sensed my frustration and asked that we have a heart-to-heart talk about it. As we talked, the obvious truth came out. The reality was this: it was easier to blame Kris than it was to admit that I (and I alone) had allowed my life to get a little out of control. The moment I realized that my frustration had everything to do with me, not Kris, everything changed.

Often when you're frustrated, this is a signal that something is going on with you. Our suggestion is this: The next time you feel angry, resentful, or frustrated by your partner or someone else, use it as an opportunity to look carefully in the mirror. What you discover may save your sanity—and your relationship.

100.

DON'T KEEP PEOPLE WAITING

One of the ways I attempt to keep my own stress under control is to avoid, whenever possible, the bad habit of keeping other people waiting. Time is precious to everyone. This being the case, one of the ultimate slaps in the face and most surefire ways to annoy someone is to keep them waiting.

While most people are somewhat forgiving, keeping them waiting is a sign of disrespect and a lack of acknowledgment. The subtle message is, "My time is more important than yours." Consider the magnitude of this suggestion. Do you feel that anyone else's time is more precious than yours? I doubt it.

It's highly stressful to keep other people waiting because you know you are disappointing someone. There are obviously exceptions to the rule—times when factors beyond your control prevent you from being on time. Truthfully, however, a vast majority of the time, being late is preventable. But instead of planning ahead, we wait just a little too long, or don't allow quite enough time—so we end up late.

When you're on time, however, you avoid all this stress and then some. You'll stop rushing and, because you won't be so hurried, you'll relax a little bit and have slightly more time to reflect.

101.

DO IT ANYWAY

I have an amazing secret that works remarkably well. It can be summed up in a single sentence that is also the title of Susan Jeffers's wonderful book: *Feel the Fear and Do It Anyway!* I've found that virtually every time I'm really frightened to do something, and I go ahead and do it anyway, it almost always turns out okay. It passes. I always survive.

Think of all the times you've lost sleep over something you had to do. A job interview, a hard conversation. You fretted and worried, but despite all the worry, you managed to get through it. Despite your fears, here you are.

This doesn't mean you haven't had difficult things to do, but it does mean that the worry we experience is nothing more than a mental irritant.

There's a lesson here for all of us. We're stronger than our fears and more competent than our worries. The next time you find yourself worrying, ask yourself: "Is it possible that I'm merely repeating a mental exercise? Do I think the worry is going to help? Aren't I going to do whatever I'm worried about anyway? What's the point of the worry?" If you take the time to reflect on these questions, you'll agree that if you "feel the fear and do it anyway," all will be well.

102.

JUMP AHEAD AND LOOK BACK

One day I was sitting with Kris at lunch when she posed the question, "Someday, when we look back on our lives together, I wonder what we will remember most and what will have been most important."

Somehow, everything appears clearer and substantially less urgent when looked at from a distance. With enough time, you're somehow able to put things in perspective and to differentiate between what's truly relevant and what only seems relevant at the moment. As you imagine looking back over your life, you can see it more objectively.

We realized that, in the end, most of the things that trouble most of us will be remembered as completely irrelevant, if they are remembered at all. Why don't we make the decision to drop our frustration now? That's what this strategy is all about—learning to drop things that you know in your heart aren't worth fretting about.

I encourage you to take some time and reflect on this exercise. Go on and jump ahead in your mind to the end of your life. Now look back and observe what you see. With any luck, you'll notice a thing or two you might consider changing—a priority, a habit, a self-defeating belief, or an attitude about life.

103.

IMAGINE THE PEOPLE IN YOUR LIFE AS TINY INFANTS AND AS ONE-HUNDRED-YEAR-OLD ADULTS

I learned this technique almost twenty years ago. It has proven to be extremely successful for releasing feelings of irritation toward other people.

Think of someone who truly irritates you, who makes you feel angry. Now, close your eyes and try to imagine this person as a tiny infant. See their tiny little features and their innocent little eyes. Know that babies can't help but make mistakes and each of us was, at one time, a little infant. Now, roll forward the clock one hundred years. See the same person as a very old person who is about to die. Look at their worn-out eyes and their soft smile, which suggests a bit of wisdom and the admission of mistakes made. Know that each of us will be one hundred years old, alive or dead, before too many decades go by.

You can play with this technique and alter it in many ways. It almost always provides the user with some needed perspective and compassion. If our goal is to become more peaceful and loving, we certainly don't want to harbor negativity toward others.

104.

CONSIDER THAT WISDOM MAY BE EVEN MORE IMPORTANT THAN IQ

While you could rank people in terms of their IQ, wisdom is a quality that you cannot accurately measure. It's invisible. Wisdom is your sense of knowing, an intuitive feeling. William James, often thought of as the "father of modern psychology," said, "Wisdom is seeing something in a nonhabitual manner." It's seeing an old problem in a new, fresh light.

One of my favorite stories that demonstrates wisdom is about a giant truck that got stuck under an overpass. The police called out the best engineers in the city to try to figure out what to do. They racked their brains for hours. Then a small boy walked up to the men and tugged on one of their pants legs. "Excuse me, sir," the little boy said in a respectful tone. "Why don't you just let the air out of the tires?" Out of the mouths of babes.

The best way to access your wisdom is simply to know that it exists and to trust in it. When you feel that your thinking is too frenetic, overactive, or that you are trying too hard, experiment with backing off. You will find that a softer focus and less effort, not more, will usually result in a better use of the mind. Relax and succeed.

105.

NEVER UNDERESTIMATE THE POWER OF LOVE

Years ago, I was at a relationship seminar when a member of the audience stood up and asked the speaker, "Why should I act loving to my wife? She doesn't act loving to me!" The speaker responded in a gentle and nonjudgmental manner. "Because you need the practice."

His words hit me like a ton of bricks and have always stuck with me. I can't think of a single person who doesn't need more practice in the art of acting loving. Can you?

With rare exception, we all need practice in unconditional love. We can all stand to be less defensive, selfish, and reactive. Most of us would be better off if we were better listeners, kinder, gentler, and a little more generous. But to embrace these qualities requires practice. It's easy to be kind and loving when our partner, friend, or child is already doing so. It's something else altogether to do so when they are not.

If you can respond with love instead of reacting with frustration and if you can keep your heart open, even when it seems unwarranted, you will have discovered the power of love and the most effective way to ensure lasting and nourishing relationships in your life. All that is required is your intention to do so, along with—you guessed it—plenty of practice.

106.

SEEK FIRST TO UNDERSTAND

This is adopted from one of Stephen Covey's "Seven Habits of Highly Effective People."

Essentially, "seek first to understand" implies that you become more interested in understanding others and less in having other people understand you. If you want quality, fulfilling communication that is nourishing to you and others, understanding others must come first. When you understand where people are coming from, what they are trying to say, what's important to them, and so forth, being understood flows naturally; it falls into place with virtually no effort. When you try to be understood before you understand, the effort you exert will be felt by you and the person or people you are trying to reach. Communication will break down, and you may end up with a battle of egos.

Seeking first to understand isn't about who's right or wrong; it is a philosophy of effective communication. When you practice this method you'll notice that the people you communicate with will feel listened to, heard, and understood. This will translate into better, more loving relationships.

107.

CREATE A BRIDGE BETWEEN YOUR SPIRITUALITY AND YOUR WORK

To create a bridge between your spirituality and your work means that you take the essence of who you are into your daily work life. You dismantle the dichotomy that exists between your spiritual life and your work. It means that if kindness, patience, and generosity are spiritual qualities that you believe in, you make every effort to practice those qualities at work.

Work is a perfect environment to practice your spirituality. In a given day, you have so many opportunities to practice patience, acts of kindness, and forgiveness. You can exhibit it in the way you sell a product—or the way you balance ethics with profit.

Grace is someone who, in my opinion, has created this bridge very well. She describes her spiritual philosophy as one of "nonviolence, integrity, and a love of all creatures." I have never seen an instance where she didn't "walk her talk." She turns down potential projects when they conflict with her values, even when she is turning away guaranteed money. I've seen her walk away from an offer when questionable ethics were involved.

There's something really comforting about creating this spiritual bridge. It reminds you of a higher purpose. It puts your problems into a broader context. It helps you grow from your difficult experiences rather than become overwhelmed by them.

108.

LEARN TO DEFLECT OCCASIONAL UNCALLED-FOR COMMENTS

There doesn't seem to be any way to get through life without saying some pretty stupid things. You're going to slip up every once in a while—when you're tired, insecure, grumpy, or just in a bad mood. Occasionally, you're likely to say something insensitive, condescending, arrogant, mean-spirited, or just plain uncalled-for. Probably all of the above. The fact is, you're human. But so are the people in your life! And humans make mistakes.

If you can make allowances for the fact that others, like you, are going to mess up every once in a while, you'll have an edge that very few seem to enjoy. What's more, your lack of insistence that your loved ones be flawless will create an emotional environment that will bring out the best in them. When someone doesn't feel pressured to be perfect, the most common response is to open the heart and act more loving.

Obviously, I'm referring to a normally healthy and loving relationship, and the way you respond to an *occasional* slip of the tongue or uncalled-for comment. We're not talking about excusing abusive behavior or *patterns* of negative behavior. But you may find that it's easier than you imagine to begin thinking of occasional uncalled-for comments as "small stuff" rather than as such a big deal.

109.

BE WILLING TO TAKE ADVICE

Generally speaking, people don't take advice, even good advice. This is true even when the advice is free and when it's offered with love. Think about yourself. How often do you really, honestly take someone else's advice?

This type of humility is almost unheard of in our culture, yet in order to grow, we need to see things differently. We don't want to do the same things over and over if they're not working well. Instead, we want to open our eyes to new and improved ways of doing things. But how can we see things differently if we refuse to take to heart the suggestions from others?

Sometimes, the reason we don't take advice is pure stubbornness. We want to do things our own way—even if it's not working! Other times, we avoid advice out of fear. We might be frightened that we're going to look bad in the eyes of someone else, or that we're going to seem incompetent.

My suggestion in this area is simple and straightforward: Take the advice. Life is so much simpler when you involve the strengths and expertise of others. After all, if you absolutely knew what to do, you'd be doing it. But if you're struggling in any aspect of your life (and we all do), you need advice.

110.

CHOOSE YOUR BATTLES WISELY

"Choose your battles wisely" is a popular phrase in parenting but is equally important in living a contented life. If you choose your battles wisely, you'll be far more effective in winning those that are truly important.

Certainly there will be times when you will want or need to argue, confront, or even fight for something you believe in. Many people, however, argue, confront, and fight over practically anything, turning their lives into a series of battles over relatively "small stuff." There are always going to be people who disagree with you, people who do things differently, and things that don't work out.

A more peaceful way to live is to decide consciously which battles are worth fighting and which are better left alone. Does your preference of which restaurant or movie to go to matter enough to argue over it? Does a small scratch on your car really warrant a suit in small claims court? Does the fact that your neighbor won't park his car on a different part of the street have to be discussed at your family dinner table? These and thousands of other small things are what many people spend their lives fighting about. Take a look at your own list.

If you don't want to "sweat the small stuff," it's critical that you choose your battles wisely.

111.

BRIGHTEN UP YOUR WORK SPACE

I wish I could have included a photograph of my office in this book. It's bright, inviting, friendly looking, and peaceful. In fact, it's so happiness-oriented that it's almost impossible to get depressed while you're in it.

Brightening up your working environment will not rid you of all your stress, nor is it the most important thing you can do to stop sweating the small stuff at work. However, you do spend an enormous amount of time where you work. Why not take a tiny bit of time, energy, and money and brighten it up, even a little?

You might be surprised at how easy it is. Try a few pictures, a brighter rug, inspirational books, freshly cut flowers, goldfish, signs of nature, or some combination. You'd be amazed at what a drawing from a child can do to lift your spirits.

I once heard the brilliant comedian Steve Martin joking about how difficult it is to feel depressed while you're playing the banjo. He was singing about death and sorrow. As he strummed the strings, it was obvious that he was right. To some extent, the same is true of your working environment. Make it bright, cheery, and friendly, and it's pretty hard to walk in and not feel the same way.

112.

DON'T COME HOME FRAZZLED

This is a simple but dramatic way to make your interactions more peaceful after a long and tiring day. It's extremely common for people to enter the home after a long day at work as if they were crossing the finish line of a race. Without even knowing it, you may be storming into the house still revved and charged from the rest of the day.

Common sense will tell you that when you're in a frantic state of mind, you are more easily agitated, annoyed, and bothered. Without even knowing it, you can be demanding, and your expectations may become elevated. Consequently, as you and your partner, children, and family engage in conversation and come together for the evening, you'll be less inclined to be fully attentive and "present."

The solution is quite simple and may take only a few minutes. Before you come home, stop your car and get out. Take a few minutes to unwind, slow down, breathe, and relax your body. Gently remind yourself that your workday is over and it's time to change gears, to slow down. What's most important is the conscious acknowledgment that it's in your best interest to be able to slow down and relax. Not only will you feel better, but your loved ones will appreciate the difference in you as well.

113.

BECOME AWARE OF YOUR MOODS AND DON'T ALLOW YOURSELF TO BE FOOLED BY LOW ONES

Your own moods can be extremely deceptive. When you're in a good mood, life looks great. You have perspective, common sense, and wisdom. But when you're in a bad mood, life looks unbearably serious and difficult. You have very little perspective.

Here's the catch: People don't realize their moods are always on the run. They think instead that their lives have suddenly become worse in the past day, or even the last hour. Such quick and drastic contrasts may seem absurd—but we're all like that. We experience the identical circumstances—who we are married to, where we work, the car we drive, our potential—entirely differently, depending on our mood!

Life is almost never as bad as it seems when you're in a low mood. Rather than staying stuck in a bad temper, convinced you are seeing life realistically, you can learn to question your judgment. Remind yourself, "Of course I'm feeling defensive [or frustrated, stressed, depressed]; I'm in a bad mood." A low mood is not the time to analyze your life. If you have a legitimate problem, it will still be there when your state of mind improves. The trick is to be grateful for our good moods and graceful in our low moods—not taking them too seriously.

114.

CONSIDER THAT BUSYNESS GETS IN YOUR WAY

Tom Hanks, one of the best actors of our time, was being interviewed on television when he responded to a question by saying, "More isn't always better." He was sharing that busyness gets in your way, that too many things going on at once can be a distraction that keeps us from being our best; when your head is too full, there's little room left for freshness and creativity.

Somewhere along the line, most of us got the message that looking, acting, and being really busy is a virtue. Certainly there are times when we truly are busy and can't do much about it. Ironically, however, when we stop worrying so much about getting everything done, when we stop looking and telling others how busy we are, we are better able to determine what's most important. We calm down and see what really needs to be done.

Schedule time in your day when absolutely nothing is going on. Even if you can only spare a few extra minutes a day, you need to have "down time." Create some space. Stop worrying that you won't get everything done. What you'll find is that when you have a little more space for yourself and a little less hurry, many of your best ideas will begin to surface.

115.

ELIMINATE THE WORRY FACTOR

There are several additional reasons to eliminate worry from your life. First and foremost, it's highly stressful. Think about how you feel when you're worried. It's all-consuming and energy-draining.

Worry is also contagious. Ellen, an ex-big-time worrier, manages a large florist. She and three other employees were preparing for a large wedding, and she was worrying more than usual. She was rushing around, visibly shaken, when she finally realized that the others were doing the same thing. They were making obvious mistakes, knocking over vases, cutting in the wrong places, and making every other mistake a florist might make.

It was obvious that her nervousness and sense of worry was indeed contagious—and that everyone around her had caught it, too. Ellen took her colleagues out for a coffee break, where everyone loosened up and relaxed. When they got back to the shop, they proceeded with their normal efficiency, not getting overly stressed about the order—and the arrangements came out perfectly.

A powerful, internal shift begins to take place as you lose your respect for worry. A new type of trust develops within yourself. In a very practical way, you begin to trust that in the absence of worry, you'll know exactly what to do and you'll know how to go about it.

116.

COMPLIMENT THE PEOPLE YOU LOVE

Ten years ago I may not have included this strategy in a book because, to me, giving compliments is as natural as brushing my teeth. I've always enjoyed giving and receiving compliments, and I married one of the most generous compliment givers imaginable. However, after discussing this topic with hundreds of people, I've come to learn that, sadly, most don't receive nearly as many compliments as they would like, particularly from their partners.

There seem to be several reasons that people don't dish out very many compliments. First, many feel as though their loved ones don't need compliments. Others simply forget how important it is. It's easy to take for granted those whom we are with a great deal of the time—so much so that their enormous contributions become invisible.

The reality is people need, thrive on, and appreciate compliments. Understand the importance of giving compliments, and begin doing so. Never assume that a compliment isn't wanted or needed. This is one of those times when more really is better. As long as your compliments are genuine and from the heart, you can't lose.

117.

GRACIOUSLY RECEIVE COMPLIMENTS

A number of years ago I was listening to a radio talk show when the guest, an expert on relationships, alluded to the fact that one of the saddest mistakes people make in relationships is the failure to receive compliments. Over the past decade, I've listened to many people receive compliments, and I, too, have come to the same conclusion.

Some of us feel a little shy, awkward, or embarrassed when someone gives us a compliment. We might respond by blushing or saying something to minimize the kind words. For example, when someone says, "You're really good at that," you might say something like, "Not really," or "I'm not as good as you think." Another way we sometimes deflect a compliment is to turn it around. So, in response to the statement, "You look really nice today," you might say, "Not as nice as you."

It takes thoughtfulness, courage, and kindness to give someone a genuine, heartfelt compliment. So, when someone rejects your compliment, however unintentionally, it hurts.

This is an easy problem to solve. The trick is to think less about what the compliment says about you—and more about what it means to the person giving it to you. When you do, you'll find it more natural to graciously receive your compliments.

118.

STAY OUT OF REVERSE

Reverse, in a psychological sense, works the same as the reverse gear in your car—it takes you backward. And, like your car, if you want to change direction and begin moving forward, you must shift gears completely.

The way reverse sounds in day-to-day living is this: "Can you believe what happened yesterday?" "Those guys were jerks." "I'm still mad at what she said to me." Anytime you are fixated on, immobilized by, or even overly concerned with something that is over—whether it happened this morning or ten years ago—constitutes reverse gear.

Take an honest look at how often you are stuck in reverse.

Obviously, it's important to learn from our past, but being stuck in reverse gear will not help you do so. If you can observe yourself, you can gently bring your attention back to the present. Training your mind to stay out of reverse can be a little like training a puppy to stay at your side. The puppy will stay for a minute, then dart away. Your mind is like that, too. As you notice your thoughts drifting backward, remind yourself that the past is over. Then, gently and easily, guide yourself back to the here and now. All it takes is a little patience and some practice.

119.

LIFE IS A TEST. IT IS ONLY A TEST.

One of my favorite posters says, "Life is a test. It is only a test. Had this been a real life, you would have been instructed where to go and what to do." Whenever I think of this humorous bit of wisdom, it reminds me to not take my life so seriously.

When you look at life and its many challenges as a test, or series of tests, you begin to see issues you face as an opportunity to grow. Whatever you're facing, when looked at as a test, you always have a chance to succeed, to rise above that which is challenging you. If you see each new issue you face as a serious battle that must be won in order to survive, you're probably in for a very rocky journey.

As an experiment, see if you can apply this idea to something you are forced to deal with. Perhaps you have a difficult teenager or a demanding boss. Redefine the issue you face from being a "problem" to being a test. Ask yourself, "Why is this issue in my life? What would it mean and what would be involved to rise above it? Could I possibly look at this issue any differently?"

If you give this strategy a try, you may be surprised at your changed responses.

120.

TAKE YOUR BREAKS

One of the worst habits I developed early on in my career was my failure to take adequate breaks. I'm a little embarrassed to admit it, but I felt they were a waste of time. I assumed that by skipping my breaks unless it was absolutely necessary, I'd be able to save a great deal of time and get more done—I'd have an edge.

I've learned that a failure to take regular breaks is an enormous mistake that not only wears you down over time but actually makes you less productive. While you may not even feel it at the time, slowly but surely your frustration will sneak up on you. You'll become less patient and attentive, and your concentration and listening skills will suffer.

Your breaks don't have to be disruptive or last very long. Usually, all you need is a few minutes to clear your head, take some deep breaths, stretch your arms, or get some air. When you take this time—every hour, or so—you'll return to your work more enthusiastic and ready to go.

This strategy reinforces the idea that more isn't always better. I feel that by working a few less minutes each hour, I'll work smarter, more efficiently, and actually get more work accomplished.

121.

AVOID ABSOLUTE STATEMENTS (OF A NEGATIVE NATURE)

Absolute statements are those that use words like *always*, *never*, *worthless*, *nothing*, and so forth. Examples of absolute statements include, "You always say the wrong thing," "You never spend any time with the kids," "Your contribution is worthless," "You do nothing to help," and so forth. Any statement that defines a person or explains contribution in a narrow, absolute way falls into this category.

There are two very important reasons to never again use these types of statements. First, as just mentioned, absolute statements can be insulting and hurtful as they are almost never accurate. Think about how you would feel if your partner said to you, "You never help around the house." In all likelihood, you'd be either hurt, annoyed, or defensive. If you had been making any effort whatsoever, your partner's words would probably be received as a stab in the back and as an untruthful jab.

The other reason it's so important not to use absolute statements is that they encourage someone to do (or not do) the very things you are objecting to. After all, you've already shared your negative perspective, so why in the world would they want to cooperate now? You're not going to give them credit, even if they do.

Whenever possible, stay away from absolute statements.

122.

BE AWARE OF POSITIVE BURNOUT

Burnout is a major topic of conversation. We discuss it, dread it, and have theories about why it exists. Virtually everyone will experience burnout at some point in their career. The most common reaction to burnout, however, is our fear surrounding it.

But have you ever stepped back far enough to see the *positive* side of burnout? Often, burnout is a signal that something new, exciting, and profitable is just around the corner!

There was a time in my life when I thought I was going to make it as a professional tennis player. Yet after many years of aches and pains, as well as some noticeable shortcomings in my game, I began to feel burned out. If not for my burnout, I would have missed out on a great education and a personally fulfilling career.

The point here is that it's not at all necessary to freak out or worry when you feel burned out.

Worry gets in the way of your wisdom and common sense. As you let go of fear, as you investigate your feelings of burnout, you may discover that your feelings are trying to tell you something, point you in a new direction, redirect your energy—or something else that is *positive* in nature.

123.

PRAISE AND BLAME ARE ALL THE SAME

One of the most unavoidable life lessons is having to deal with the disapproval of others. Even in a "landslide" election victory in which a candidate secures 55 percent of the vote, he or she is left with the knowledge that 45 percent of the population wishes someone else were the winner. Pretty humbling, isn't it?

Our approval rating from family, friends, and the people we work with isn't likely to be much higher. The truth is, everyone has their own set of ideas with which to evaluate life, and our ideas don't always match those of other people. We get angry, hurt, or otherwise frustrated when people reject our ideas, tell us no, or give us some other form of disapproval.

The sooner we accept the inevitable dilemma of not being able to win the approval of everyone we meet, the easier our lives will become. When you expect to be dished out your share of disapproval, you'll develop a helpful perspective to assist your life journey.

There are many days when I experience both praise and blame. Someone will hire me to speak, and someone else won't; one phone call delivers good news, another announces a new issue to deal with. This back-and-forth, good and bad, approval and disapproval, is a part of everyone's life.

124.

DON'T TAKE THE 80/20 RULE PERSONALLY

According to the 80/20 rule, in the workplace, 20 percent of the people do approximately 80 percent of the work.

I've observed that many "overachievers" don't even see themselves as achievers—but rather as ordinary people who simply do what it takes to succeed or get the job done. I knew a superachieving man who insisted, "I'm not an overachiever. It's just that most people are underachievers." He wasn't intentionally being arrogant; he genuinely saw things this way.

You may not have such an extreme vision (I certainly don't), but you too may find it hard to accept (or understand) that other people have different priorities, work ethics, gifts, and mind-sets. Remember, different people also define productivity in very different ways.

Try paying less attention to what other people aren't doing, and put more emphasis on what you get out of your own level of productivity—financially, energetically, emotionally, even spiritually. You are not a victim of others who make different choices, or who, for whatever reason, aren't as productive as you, at least according to your standards.

I encourage you to examine your own expectation that others work like you do. Accept the fact that it's not personal, and you can lighten up enough to appreciate the differences in people and the way they choose to work.

125.

PRACTICE RANDOM ACTS OF KINDNESS

There is a bumper sticker that has been around for some time now that reads "Practice Random Acts of Kindness and Senseless Acts of Beauty." I have no idea who thought of this idea, but I've never seen a more important message on a car in front of me. Practicing random kindness is an effective way to get in touch with the joy of giving without expecting anything in return. It's best practiced without letting anyone know what you are doing.

There are five toll bridges in the San Francisco Bay Area. A while back, some people began paying the tolls of the cars immediately behind them. The drivers would drive to the toll window only to be informed, "Your toll has been paid by the car ahead of you." This is an example of a spontaneous, random gift, something given without expectation of or demand for anything in return.

There is no prescription for how to practice random kindness. It comes from the heart. Perhaps the greatest reason to practice random kindness is that it brings great contentment into your life. Each act of kindness rewards you with positive feelings and reminds you of the important aspects of life—service, kindness, and love.

126.

DIVE IN

If you're going to do something important, the best time to start is right now. Not later, tomorrow, next week, next month, or next year. Right now. The best strategy is to "dive in." I know there's always an important reason to put off doing today what you are planning or hoping to do tomorrow. In fact, there are usually many good reasons to wait. Despite these good reasons, however, I urge you to get started now.

About a year ago I and Kris attended a meeting designed to help kick-start new businesses. There was a bright and talented woman in the audience. This woman decided to wait. Despite being "certain" (her word) that she wanted to get involved, she wanted to "think about it" for a while. She wanted the time to be right.

A few months later, we attended a different meeting where my wife was one of the speakers. Who did we see? The same woman. We urged her to get started. "Not quite yet" was her response. She was "really committed" to the program but didn't want to "dive in" (again, her words).

The secret to success is to understand that, despite everything, the best time to begin is now. You don't have to do everything in one day to succeed, but you do have to get started.

127.

MAKE A PLAN TO BECOME MORE LOVING

It's extremely helpful to have a well-thought-out plan in place to ensure that you will become a more loving person. I'm not talking about creating a plan in order to get more love or to manipulate someone into loving you, but one designed to help you become the most loving person that you can become.

Whenever you want to go from A to Z, it's almost always easier if you have a plan.

Having a plan—short-term goals and long-term goals—and working toward those goals usually pays enormous dividends in terms of becoming the type of person you want to become.

When I first met Steve, he was a nice guy but, in his words, "more than a little uptight"—reactive and tense, and almost always in a hurry. However, he had a sincere goal—and a long-term plan—to become a more loving human being. He worked daily on his listening skills. He read books with differing points of view and practiced patience and gratitude. He took courses on communication and relationship skills, and he mastered several techniques on stress reduction.

We all have the capacity to change and to become the people we want to be. Having a plan in place can help us make those changes and bring them to life, whatever they happen to be, and makes our journey seem more manageable. Good luck.

128.

MAKE A LIST OF YOUR PERSONAL PRIORITIES

I'll warn you in advance that this strategy can be humbling, but ultimately very helpful. It involves taking a careful look at those personal things that you feel are most important to you. Once you decide what they are, write them down on a sheet of paper and put the list away for a week or two.

Here's the hard part: after some time has gone by, take out your list and read it to yourself. Now, think back honestly, how have you spent your free time? If your actions over the past few weeks were consistent with your list, congratulations!

If, however, you look at your list and realize (as I did) that a staggering percentage of your time was spent doing other things, then you've got work to do. To varying degrees, we ignore that which we insist is more important in favor of things that seem pressing or are simply more convenient.

A friend of mine said, "In reality, you vote with your actions, not your words." This means that while I can tell you that my friends and family are important to me, ultimately, the measure of what's most important to me is how I spend my time and energy.

You have the power to implement your priorities.

129.

LOOK BEYOND BEHAVIOR

Have you ever heard yourself, or someone else, say: "Don't mind John, he didn't know what he was doing"? If so, you have been exposed to the wisdom of "looking beyond behavior." If you have children, you know very well the importance of this simple act of forgiveness. If our love for our children was based on their behavior, it would often be difficult to love them at all.

Wouldn't it be nice if we could try to extend this same loving-kindness toward everyone we meet? Wouldn't we live in a more loving world if, when someone acted in a way that we didn't approve of, we could see their actions in a similar light as our teenagers' offbeat behavior?

This doesn't mean that we walk around with our heads in the sand, pretend that everything is always wonderful, or that we excuse or approve of bad behavior. Instead, it simply means having the perspective to give others the benefit of the doubt. When your spouse or close friend snaps at you, try to understand that, beneath this isolated act, your loved one really wants to love you and to feel loved by you. Looking beyond behavior is easier than you might think. Try it today, and you'll see and feel some nice results.

130.

JUST ONCE, TRY SOMETHING DIFFERENT

Many of us do the same things, day after day, for most of our adult lives. We have the same habits, go to the same places, hold the same opinions, get upset over the same things, think the same thoughts, meet with the same people, do things in the same way. How boring!

Most people are stuck right where they are. The reason they're stuck, however, isn't usually due to circumstances or lack of opportunity, but a simple unwillingness to change, to try new things.

I'm referring here to smaller, inner changes that you can make on a day-to-day, moment-to-moment basis—changes in your attitude, reactions, and expectations. I'm talking about being willing to meet new people at new places, take new risks, and face old fears. Perhaps you can, for once, listen to someone else's opinion or read a news source that you usually disagree with.

Starting today, tell yourself that you are going to do something, however small, a little differently. Perhaps you can be more friendly to the people you work with. Maybe it's not too late to overcome your fear of asking others to help you or for their advice. Experiment with newness. Just once, try something different.

131.

SEE THE INNOCENCE

For many people, one of the most frustrating aspects of life is not being able to understand other people's behavior. We see them as "guilty" instead of "innocent." It's tempting to focus on people's seemingly irrational behavior—their comments, actions, selfish behavior—and get extremely frustrated.

But as I once heard Wayne Dyer sarcastically suggest in a lecture, "Round up all the people who are making you miserable and bring them to me. I will treat them [as a counselor], and you'll get better!" Obviously, this is absurd. It's true that other people do weird things (who doesn't?), but *we* are the ones getting upset, so we are the ones who need to change. I'm not talking about accepting, ignoring, or advocating violence or any other deviant behavior. I'm merely talking about learning to be less *bothered* by the actions of others.

Seeing the innocence is a powerful tool for transformation that means when someone is acting in a way that we don't like, the best strategy for dealing with that person is to distance ourselves from the behavior; to "look beyond it," so that we can see the innocence in where the behavior is coming from.

The next time (and hopefully from now on) someone frustrates you, look for the innocence. If you're compassionate, it won't be hard to see.

132.

GRACEFULLY ACCEPT APOLOGIES

Sadly, many people find it difficult to apologize. One of the reasons this might be true is because, when we do apologize, it's often accepted in a less than graceful manner. When this is the case, it takes some of the motivation away to continue apologizing, even when appropriate.

I overheard what I thought was an excellent example of this problem while I was sitting at a coffee shop. With tears in her eyes, a woman was sharing with her husband that she was sorry that her work had become so consuming. Obviously, I don't know all the facts, and they certainly aren't any of my business. However, regardless of the specifics, one thing was perfectly clear. His inability to soften and open his heart in response to her genuine and heartfelt apology was guaranteeing an escalation of any problems they were already having.

In order for an apology to be effective, both parties must do their part. When apologies aren't accepted, bitterness and resentment often creep into the picture. We've found that, in most instances, an apology is an excellent opportunity to deepen a relationship. It's an ideal time to make a genuine effort to listen deeply and respectfully.

The next time someone offers an apology, see if you can really take it to heart. Soften your edges and open your heart.

133.

HELP SOMEONE ELSE SUCCEED

It's been said that the absolute best way to learn something is to try to teach it. Teaching others helps us pinpoint our knowledge and the way we express it. It encourages us to think in creative, articulate ways. We want to practice in our own lives what we teach.

There are probably many people in your life you are in a position to help. Perhaps you're very experienced in your field. Maybe there is someone who could use some feedback, advice, or encouragement. Is there someone in your family or circle of friends who is struggling? If you look around, I'll bet you can find someone who would really appreciate your help.

I'm not suggesting that you overwhelm someone with your presence or with your ideas. Be sure to get permission before offering your help. Be gentle and patient. Not everyone wants or is ready for help. And that's okay. Don't take it personally.

As you help others succeed, even in very small ways, it helps you redefine and reflect on your own goals, assumptions, and ways of doing things. I'm often amazed at how my advice applies to my own life. Recently, someone asked me for advice. Upon reflection, I suggested that he desperately needed a break or else he might burn out. And I realized that *I* needed to slow down too!

134.

CHOOSE BEING KIND OVER BEING RIGHT

As I first introduced on day 46, you are given many opportunities to choose between being kind and being right. These opportunities amount to chances to make someone else feel bad, and to make yourself feel bad in the process.

The reason we are tempted to put others down, correct them, or show them how we're right and they're wrong is that our ego mistakenly believes that if we point out how someone else is wrong, we must be right, and therefore we will feel better.

In actuality, however, if you pay attention to the way you feel after you put someone down, you'll notice that you feel worse than before the put-down. The compassionate part of you knows that it's impossible to feel better at the expense of someone else.

Luckily, the opposite is true—when your goal is to build people up, to share in their joy, you too reap the rewards of their positive feelings. The next time you have the chance to correct someone, even if their facts are a little off, resist the temptation. Instead, ask yourself, "What do I really want out of this interaction?" Chances are, what you want is a peaceful interaction. Each time you resist "being right" and instead choose kindness, you'll notice a peaceful feeling within.

135.

USE EFFECTIVE LISTENING AS A STRESS-REDUCING TOOL

The reason I return to listening so often is that, in my opinion, it's one of the most important ingredients for success in virtually all aspects of life—personal and professional. Unfortunately, it's also one of our greatest weaknesses.

Take a moment to reflect on your own listening skills at work. Do you truly listen to your colleagues? In meetings, are you patient and responsive—or are you impatient and reactive? Do you allow words from others to sink in, or do you assume you know what the person is trying to say, so you jump in? Simply asking yourself these and related questions can be enormously helpful.

Effective listening is an excellent stress-reducing technique. People who listen well are highly respected and sought after. Since effective listeners are loved by the people they work with (and the people they live with), they avoid many of the most common stressful aspects of work—backstabbing, resentment, sabotage, and ill feelings.

Effective listening helps you to understand what people are saying the first time they say it, thus allowing you to avoid stressful mistakes and misinterpretations.

This is one of those powerful strategies that can generate immediate and significant results. You may have to work at it a little, but if you do, it will be well worth it.

136.

PERSEVERE

When I was just getting started in business, my father said something to me that, at first, sounded a little superficial—but he was right. He told me that part of being successful was just hanging in there and sticking with it. He said that many people quit too early, get impatient, fail to defer any gratification, and move around too much.

My wife, Kris, works in a networking business that serves as an excellent example. She knows that virtually anyone can be successful in her business, but that most people fail to give it a fair try. If they have one or two disappointments early on (which most do), they allow their fear or impatience to enter into the equation, and they're on to something else. In a nutshell, they quit too early. They lack perseverance. Any new venture that is destined for success is going to take work and perseverance. If it didn't, your success wouldn't be as rewarding.

I've found that there is a delicate balance between being willing to stick something out and a willingness to make changes. You need the wisdom to know when to quit and when to stay right where you are. So, if you feel like quitting, don't do so impulsively. Instead, check in with your wisdom. If you're quitting too early, remind yourself to persevere.

137.

DON'T QUESTION THEIR MOTIVES

One of the nicest things about growing up is that you are free, within reason, to make your own decisions. There is something so nourishing and rewarding about making a choice and feeling supported in it. It's something else altogether, however, if you have to explain or defend your decision. Instead of feeling unconditionally supported, you feel as though you're on trial.

I overheard a woman telling her husband she was going to have lunch with an old girlfriend. His response speaks to the essence of this strategy. In a condescending tone, he said, "Why are you going to spend your time with her?" He clearly disapproved and was questioning her motives. In a matter of seconds, they went from having a relaxing afternoon to having a stressful interaction.

Questioning the motives of your partner or friends sends the message that you don't respect or approve of their decisions. It encourages highly defensive reactions and takes much of the joy out of sharing. Obviously, I'm not talking about *never* questioning a motive. If it is something that involves you or is truly crucial, that's a different matter. This is for small stuff, daily stuff.

It's so enjoyable to share with someone who allows you to do so freely, without question. If you give this a try, you'll be forever glad you did.

138.

TELL THREE PEOPLE (TODAY) HOW MUCH YOU LOVE THEM

Author Stephen Levine asks the question, "If you had an hour to live and could make only one phone call—who would you call, what would you say, and why are you waiting?" What a powerful message!

Who knows what we are waiting for? Perhaps we want to believe we will live forever, or that "someday" we will get around to telling the people we love how much we love them.

As fate would have it, I'm writing this on my grandmother's birthday. She died about two years ago. Before she passed away, it became obvious how important it was to her to let her family know how much she loved us all. Now is the time to let people know how much you care.

Ideally, you can tell someone in person or over the phone. I wonder how many people have received a call where the caller says, "I just called to tell you how much I love you!" You may be surprised that almost nothing in the world means so much to a person.

If you're too shy to make such a phone call, write a heartfelt letter instead. Either way, you may find that as you get used to it, letting people know how much you love them will become a regular part of your life.

139.

CONSIDER THE WISDOM OF OPTIMISM

There are essentially two types of people: optimists and pessimists. Which is wiser? Pessimists, of course, will tell you that they are being "realists." They insist that life is hard, things often don't work out, and it's not a good idea to set yourself up for disappointment.

It should come as no surprise to you that pessimists experience far more disappointments than optimists. The reason is simple: they are looking for failure.

Optimists, however, understand that no one has a crystal ball and that no one can accurately predict the future. Optimists believe that because no one *really* knows what's going to happen, it's far wiser and makes for a more pleasant and joyful experience of life if one assumes the best.

Your energy follows your attention. We create what we see and what we expect to see. If we have negative expectations, we will tend to create negative results. When you're looking for positive answers and expect to find them, you usually do. Does this mean you'll always succeed? Absolutely not. But unlike the pessimist who will say, "See, what did I tell you? People are difficult and stubborn," the optimist will simply chalk it up as another learning experience. There is a great deal of wisdom and joy in optimism. Give it a try.

140.

PRACTICE HUMILITY

Humility and inner peace go hand in hand. The less compelled you are to try to prove yourself to others, the easier it is to feel peaceful inside.

Proving yourself is a dangerous trap. It takes an enormous amount of energy to be continually pointing out your accomplishments, bragging, or trying to convince others of your worth as a human being.

The way to develop genuine humility is to practice it. It's nice because you will get immediate inner feedback in the way of calm, easy feelings. The next time you have an opportunity to brag, resist the temptation.

I discussed this strategy with a client, and he shared this story: He was with a group of friends a few days after he had been promoted. He was chosen to be promoted over another friend of theirs. He was a little competitive with this person and had the very strong temptation to slip in the fact that he had been chosen, and their other friend wasn't. A little voice inside him said, *"Stop. Don't do it!"* He went ahead and shared about the promotion, but didn't cross the line and mention the friend who wasn't promoted. He told me that he couldn't remember ever feeling so calm and proud of himself. He was able to enjoy his success without bragging.

141.

FINISH THE JOB

For several months, Rachel had been looking forward to catching up with some old friends. With three kids and busy work schedules, it was tricky to find a time that worked, but her husband, Rick, rearranged some work obligations so he could be home with the kids. Rachel had a great time reconnecting with her friends. Her heart sank, however, the moment she walked in the door. The house looked like a bomb had gone off. Rather than being able to go to bed refreshed, she came home and started cleaning up messes.

This is a sad story because Rick had gone to some lengths to be there. However, his lack of effort—his unwillingness to finish the job—turned what would have been a wonderful and relaxing evening into a disappointment!

In this story, "finishing the job" meant cleaning up. But it just as easily could have been making the phone calls that you promised you would make, delivering on a promise, or making a dinner reservation. It's really that simple.

There are plenty of exceptions to this rule. There are times when you just can't do things—you're either too exhausted or too busy, or you just plain forgot. However, the moral of the story is this: Whenever possible and within reason, try to go the extra mile for your loved ones.

142.

HOLD ON TIGHTLY, LET GO LIGHTLY

"Hold on tightly, let go lightly" is a motto that encourages you to obtain the optimal balance between productivity and inner peace. "Hold on" suggests that you want to work hard, stick with things, persevere, and pursue your goals. The "let go lightly" side, however, suggests that you shouldn't hold on too long, and that when it is time to give in, give up, or let go, that you do so gracefully.

An excellent example of holding on tightly and letting go lightly exists in parenting. When we raise our children, most of us want to hold on tightly when they're young. We work very hard to protect them, to expose them to varied experiences. We defend their safety and their honor. But then there comes a time when you need to "let go," when you need to set them free, to step aside and allow them to live their own lives. Letting go has nothing to do with ceasing to love our children. In fact, letting go is one of the ultimate expressions of a parent's love.

When the time does come to say goodbye, or to make a change in life, try doing so with grace. This will keep you pointed in the direction of your dreams. Instead of looking back, you'll be focused on your next great adventure.

143.

MAKE FRIENDS WITH EVERYONE

Not too long ago I was in San Francisco in a reception lounge, waiting for my lunch partner.

A man walked in and barked out, in a demanding tone, "Any messages?" The female receptionist looked up and replied pleasantly back saying there were none. He responded in a nasty, almost threatening manner, "Be sure to call me when my twelve-thirty appointment arrives. Got it?" He stormed down the hall.

Shortly after, a woman entered the room. She smiled, said "hello," and asked the receptionist about her day. The receptionist smiled back and thanked the woman for asking. She gave the woman her mail and chatted. They laughed together a few times before the woman thanked the receptionist and walked down the hall.

The difference between those two quick interactions was striking, and it no doubt impacted how all three of those people felt that day.

My suggestion is to think of your receptionist, the folks in the mail room, the administrative assistants, IT, the office manager, and any other people in supporting roles as key partners in your life. Treat them as if you truly value them—as you should. Be kind, genuine, patient, and courteous. Thank them when they do something for you—even if it's part of their job. Their work is important and too often invisible to those around them.

144.

BE WILLING TO APOLOGIZE

Many people never apologize. They are either too self-conscious, self-righteous, stubborn, or arrogant to do so. But almost everyone expects others to make mistakes. And with a humble and sincere apology, almost everyone is willing to forgive.

On a live television talk show once I was discussing one of my books. I was in a terrible mood, and my interaction with a guest asking for advice ended up hurting his feelings. The producer contacted me telling me that as far as she was concerned, I wasn't welcome on her show again! Instead of being defensive, I offered my most sincere apology. I told her that I was wrong and that she was right. I really meant what I said.

A few weeks went by, and I received another letter from the producer. She said that in over ten years as a producer, she had never received such a sincere and nondefensive apology. She asked if I would come back as a guest again real soon.

I tell you this story to remind you of how forgiving people can be when you admit you're wrong. When you apologize from your heart, you keep most of your existing doors open. Occasionally, you may even open doors that had previously been closed.

145.

ASK A LOVED ONE, "WHAT'S THE MOST DIFFICULT PART OF BEING IN A RELATIONSHIP WITH ME?"

It's understandable that, for many people, this can be a somewhat frightening experience. The fear, of course, lies in discovering what you might find out—or what someone might say to you, given the permission to speak their mind.

This strategy does require an openness as well as courage and humility. Despite any initial discomfort you may feel, the question tends to bring forth openness, insightful communication, and ultimately a feeling of gratitude. This is a true shortcut to better relationships.

It's interesting to observe what happens to another person's dissatisfaction when you allow, even encourage, them the privilege of getting whatever it is that concerns them off their chest. Often, when you sincerely and nondefensively want to know the answer, it will take the edge or "sting" off of the issue.

Experiment with this strategy. It may bring up something minor or something more serious. Either way, you'll get it out in the open in a nondefensive environment and you'll have the chance to make whatever it is a "nonissue." If all goes well, perhaps your loved one may even ask you for your feedback as well. If that turns out not to be the case, however, that's okay, too. Whatever you do, don't demand reciprocation.

146.

WHEN IN DOUBT ABOUT WHOSE TURN IT IS TO TAKE OUT THE TRASH, GO AHEAD AND TAKE IT OUT

If we're not careful, it's easy to become resentful about all the responsibilities of daily living.

It's astounding to me how easy it is for me to remember all the chores that I do, as well as all the other responsibilities that I take care of. But at the same time, it's easy for me to forget all the things that my wife does on a daily basis. How convenient!

It's difficult to become a contented person if you're keeping score of every chore and responsibility. It's the epitome of "small stuff." It will bring you far more joy in your life to know that you have done your part and someone else in your family has one less thing to do than it will to fret over whose turn it is to take out the trash.

The argument against this strategy is that you'll be taken advantage of. This mistake is similar to believing it's important that you're right. Most of the time it's *not* important that you're right, and neither is it important if you take out the trash more often than your spouse or housemate. Making things like garbage less relevant in your life will free up more time and energy for truly important things.

147.

IF YOU FIND YOURSELF IN A HOLE, STOP DIGGING

The great football coach Vince Lombardi once said, "Just because you're doing something wrong, doing it more intensely won't help." What a powerful statement.

Yet, how often do we do just that? We are making a mistake, and, instead of backing off, reflecting, and doing it differently, we roll up our sleeves and do the very same thing even more intensely!

This pattern exists in many areas of our lives. Many people have a great deal of conflict to manage. Whenever a potential new conflict arises, instead of looking for new ways to defuse the situation, they charge straight ahead, as always—repeating their identical patterns and responses, taking the adversarial approach—and, once again, find themselves in the middle of another drama or conflict. This is the essence of being in a vicious circle.

The solution is simple but not always very easy. The trick is to recognize when your part of the pattern is being repeated; for example, "Here I am, arguing again," or "I'm upset by the very same things—this sure feels familiar." Then, rather than clenching your fists, feeling frustrated, filling your mind with stressful thoughts, and trying the same old thing, you instead relax, back off, and empty your mind. Soften and try to see the situation in a whole new way.

148.

REMEMBER THE MOTTO, "YOU CATCH MORE FLIES WITH HONEY"

When I see someone acting aggressively or intimidating someone, pushing their weight around, or being manipulative, I feel like reminding them that, in the long run, you really do catch more flies with honey. Simply put, it pays to be nice!

When you are kind, loving, and patient—when you are fair, a good listener, and when you genuinely care about others—your attitude comes across in all you do. As a result, people love to be around you and will be comfortable in your presence. They delight in your success.

It's unfortunate, but the opposite is also true. I've met many people who have said something like, "I'll never hire that person again." When I've asked, "Weren't you happy with his work?" they will usually say, "Absolutely. That's not it at all. It's just that he is so difficult to work with."

It's important to consider this strategy even if you feel you are a relatively gentle person. Most of us—certainly I include myself—have a long way to go. Without even realizing it, we may still push others around, act a little arrogant, or use other tools of manipulation to get our way. When we reflect on the practical, real-life importance of being gentle and patient, we can become even more so.

149.

DON'T BE AFRAID TO TAKE BABY STEPS

Often, people worry about taking baby steps. They worry that the steps they are taking aren't big enough or significant enough. Or they worry that others will laugh at them or see them as weak. Many people are so frightened to take baby steps that they end up doing nothing at all.

I've had many people ask me the best way to write a book. My answer is almost always the same: just start writing. Don't wait. Even if you can only write a single paragraph, even a sentence, it's far better than nothing. There is a common misconception that if you wait to begin, someday you'll wake up with tremendous inspiration and take a giant step. I can assure you that this *is* possible, and it can happen to you. However, you greatly increase the likelihood of taking "giant steps" if you begin with baby steps.

My wife and I decided a number of years ago to run a marathon together (yes, I'm proud of this). Our training began with twenty minutes of jogging per day—baby steps. It would have been crazy for us to wait to start our training program until we were able to run an hour. We never would have been able to do it; we needed our baby steps to succeed.

Every process, be it personal or professional, begins with baby steps.

150.

BECOME LOWER MAINTENANCE

There are two types of houseguests. The first might be called "high maintenance." These are guests who show up and take over your life. They require lots of attention and need to be constantly entertained. The other type can be called "low maintenance." You spend plenty of time together, laughing and sharing, yet, in some ways you don't even know they are there.

A very similar distinction can be made in more intimate relationships. High-maintenance individuals are usually demanding and needy, requiring lots of attention. They are frequently upset, and they need to be entertained. On the other end of the spectrum are the low-maintenance people. These are individuals who are easy to be with in every sense of the word. They are seldom needy or demanding and are sensitive to the fact that they are not the center of the universe.

Most of us, of course, fall somewhere in between. No one is completely maintenance-free, and luckily, very few people are at the other extreme, either. It's inevitable that some of the qualities of a high-maintenance person are going to show up from time to time in every relationship—it certainly does in mine. No big deal! Wherever you happen to fall on the scale is perfectly fine. However, if you make some minor changes, your loved ones will begin to notice and appreciate them.

151.

REMIND YOURSELF THAT LIFE ISN'T YOUR ENEMY, YOUR THINKING IS

At times, it can seem like life is our enemy, as if things never quite pan out the way we would like them to, as if there's a secret conspiracy against us. However, it's critical to remember that, in reality, life *isn't* our enemy. There is no conspiracy. Life is just life. It is what it is. The factor that can make life *seem* like our enemy, however, is our thinking. Nothing more, nothing less. Life wants you to succeed just as much as it does the next person.

As obvious as this insight may seem, the implications are enormous. The truth is, life isn't going to accommodate any of us by giving us fewer demands, less traffic, people who are easier to get along with, or a smoother path toward success. If we want a different experience of life, a more peaceful outlook, we are the ones who must change.

The good news, of course, is you do have a fair measure of control over your own thinking. You can change the way you think, and you can change your reactions to life. It's entirely up to you. You have the power to become anything you want to become. But to do so, you must realize that life is not your enemy; it's your friend.

152.

DON'T LIVE FOR RETIREMENT

Knowingly or unknowingly, many people practically live for retirement. They think about how wonderful life will be without the burden of daily work outside the home. Some people go so far as to count the years, months, even days before retirement. It's common for people to postpone joy, contentment, and satisfaction until "later." It's almost as though people are "doing time," or serving a sentence, patiently waiting for their freedom.

Admittedly, most people don't go quite this far. It's usually a bit more subtle than this. However, a staggering percentage of people expect that life down the road is going to be better than it is today.

I'm passionate about this topic because it's clear to me that thinking in these "someday life will be better" terms is a guaranteed way to set yourself up for a long and tiring ride. It's far better, I believe, to wake up each morning and remind yourself of the adage "Today is the first day of the rest of my life." Make the decision to honor your gift of life by giving today your best effort.

Plan ahead and plan well. But do yourself a great big favor. Don't miss a single day along the way.

153.

DO IT YOUR WAY

Every relationship is unique. We're all different. Each of us brings to our relationships our own history, plans, fears, dreams, disappointments, and expectations. We're attracted and drawn to different things and are bugged by certain others. We've all had at least some painful experiences that shape our personality and, hopefully, many happy ones as well.

Yet many of us have the tendency to act as if our relationships—with our romantic partners, friends, and family—need to fit into a certain mold, that we have to be like everyone else. This is unfortunate because doing so can create a barrier between what you know is true for you and how you choose to live your life. It can also prevent you from following your own bliss and from discovering great joy. It can adversely affect your relationships in many ways—from the very mundane (e.g., attending parties you don't really want to go to) to the very serious (e.g., what religion you feel you must practice to keep peace in the family).

It's easy to get caught in the trap of comparing your relationship to that of others or to worry about expectations. Joyful relationships, however, are ones that you create—and that are uniquely yours. I hope you'll honor your own way and discover what works best for you.

154.

STOP SWEATING THE SMALL RISKS

Often, without even knowing we are doing so, we make a big deal out of relatively small risks. We treat small risks like big risks. And by doing that, we pay a huge price.

Some decisions really would be quite risky. Gambling with your kids' college savings fund, of course, would be extremely risky. Screaming at your employer would be risky, as would driving without a seat belt!

There are many other activities, however, that we tend to worry about, often obsessively, that maybe we shouldn't. Things like asking for a raise, whether or not to take certain advice, or worrying about how someone will react to us. These activities may, in fact, frighten us, but there is very little actual risk associated with them. The cost of treating these things like big risks is exceptionally high.

It can be quite helpful to create a list of truly legitimate risks, things that could adversely affect your life. You'll probably find that the list you create is going to be quite short. Next, jot down the more subtle things that you tend to worry about. You'll probably create a much longer list of these perceived risks. When you see the "real" risks next to the others, right there on paper, it's often easier to convince yourself to let go of the ones that are less severe.

155.

SPEND A MOMENT, EVERY DAY, THINKING OF SOMEONE TO LOVE

Earlier in this book I introduced the idea of spending a moment, every day, thinking of someone to thank. Another excellent source of gratitude is to spend a moment, every day, thinking of someone to love.

I started consciously choosing to think of people to love when I realized how often I could get caught up in thinking about the opposite—people who irritate me. Once I made the conscious decision, however, to spend a moment each morning thinking of someone to love, my attention was redirected toward the positive, not only toward that one person, but in general throughout the day. I don't mean to suggest that I never get irritated anymore, but without question it happens much less frequently than it used to.

Every morning when I wake up, I close my eyes and ask myself the question, "Who shall I send love to today?" Instantly, a picture of someone will pop into my mind, and I simply wish them a day filled with love. Those few seconds stick with me for many hours. If you give this little exercise a try, I think you'll find that your day is a little more peaceful.

156.

WAKE UP AND THINK ABOUT THREE THINGS YOU LOVE

At the risk of sounding corny, this strategy really works. I've found that it's nearly impossible to get too uptight or to sweat the small stuff with your loved ones when you have recently reminded yourself about why you love them so much. This holds true whether you're thinking about a romantic partner, family members, friends, or your kids.

A few days ago I woke up and thought about the way Kris brightens the lives of others with her beautiful smile. For as long as I can remember, she's been smiling and being nice to everyone, even strangers. I don't think I've ever picked her up at the airport when she didn't have a new friend she had met on the plane! This led me to two more loving thoughts in quick succession. The entire process probably took about a minute or two, but it set the stage for the rest of the day.

This doesn't mean that if you think about several things you appreciate about your loved ones, first thing every morning, that you're never again going to become irritated or annoyed. It will, however, substantially reduce the likelihood of this occurring. This strategy is quick, simple, effective, and virtually effortless. What's more, it feels good.

157.

AVOID THE PHRASE, "I HAVE TO GO TO WORK"

I'm going to suggest a strategy that has to do with six of the most common words in the English language: "I have to go to work." Before I continue, let me assure you that I'm aware that, in all probability, it's absolutely true that you do have to go to work. Nevertheless, these particular words carry with them some really negative baggage.

Other than your thoughts, your words are your primary entry point into your experience. They paint a picture of your expectation and pave the way toward your experience. When you "have" to do something, it implies that it's not a choice—that you'd rather be somewhere else, doing something different. So, when you say, "I have to go to work," you're subtly setting yourself up for a bad day.

It seems that deep down, what you're really saying is, "I don't like my work. I'm not capable of choosing work that I enjoy." What a horrible message to say to yourself about something you spend most of your time doing!

I think you're going to be surprised at what may happen if you change your words. Why not get yourself off to a good start by avoiding the tendency to bad-mouth what you are about to do?

158.

HAVE A PLAN

It's quite difficult to get somewhere if you don't know where you're headed. Yet a huge percentage of us have no plan. We don't really know where we're going or how we're going to get there. It's easy to look and feel extremely busy when we don't have a plan, but in reality we're just spinning our wheels, putting out fires, or chasing our tails.

When you have a predetermined plan, something magical happens: Your plan helps you to draw out your inner strength, creativity, and discipline. In some mysterious way, you are usually able to stick to your plan once you have one in place.

With a plan in mind, the sky's the limit. As long as you can visualize a way to implement your plan, your dreams—however big—can become a reality. Your plan may be to become a multimillionaire, to run a marathon, or to spend an extra day each week with your children. It doesn't matter what your plan is, but it does matter that you have one. Make a plan today.

159.

DON'T GET LOST IN YOUR PLAN

One of my favorite quotes is "Life is what's happening while we're busy making other plans." Many people get lost in their dreams of becoming successful. So much so that they sacrifice their relationships with family members, friends, even themselves. They are focused on the result, not on the steps along the way. The steps, however, are where you find the joy.

When people become obsessed with their plans, it is often because they worry too much about their success and the direction of their lives. Keep in mind that worrying interferes with your ability to create abundance; it gets in the way and clouds your vision. When you stop worrying, your plan will have a chance to unfold.

Keep in touch with your sense of knowing, that inner awareness that any goal or dream you have, as long as you know what it is, is within your grasp. An important aspect of a successful life is balancing these two seemingly different messages (having a plan, but not getting lost in it). My advice is to know exactly where you'd like to go and exactly how you plan to get there. But at the same time, let go of your goal and enjoy the ride. Each step of your journey is an important part of your unique curriculum.

160.

STAY AWAY FROM COMPARISONS

Shortly after my first child was born, Kris and I were having dinner with friends. At some point during the evening our friend Cassie said to several others, "I wish David (her husband) would spend more time with our children like Richard does." Her husband overheard and was furious.

As is almost always the case, the comparison was ludicrous and unfair, like apples and oranges. I was self-employed and have a short commute, while David had very little control over his schedule and an hour plus commute.

I'm certain that our friend meant no harm by her comment. She was merely expressing her frustration that David couldn't spend more time with the kids, and thought it was nice that I was able to do so. Unfortunately, however, that innocent and legitimate explanation was meaningless. Once you compare someone who loves you to someone else, you've opened the door for potential trouble.

There is another side of the coin to be aware of as well. If you're on the receiving end of a comparison, try not to "sweat it." Instead, try to see the innocence in the comment and let it go.

We've yet to meet someone who appreciates being compared (in a deficient sort of way) to someone else. Nor do we expect to any time soon. Comparisons are indeed something we should all stay away from.

161.

BECOME AN ANTHROPOLOGIST

Anthropology is a science dealing with man and his origins. In this strategy, however, I'll conveniently redefine anthropology as "being interested, without judgment, in the way other people choose to live and behave." This strategy is geared toward developing your compassion, as well as a way of becoming more patient. Being interested in the way other people act is a way of replacing judgments with loving-kindness. When you are genuinely curious about the way someone reacts or the way they feel about something, it's unlikely that you will also be annoyed.

When someone acts in a way that seems strange to you, rather than reacting in your usual way, such as, "I can't believe they would do that," instead say something to yourself like "I see, that must be the way she sees things in her world. Very interesting." In order for this strategy to help you, you have to be genuine. There's a fine line between being "interested" and being arrogant, as if secretly you believe that your way is better.

When you are interested in other perspectives, it doesn't imply, even slightly, that you're advocating it. One of the cardinal rules of joyful living is that judging others takes a great deal of energy and, without exception, pulls you away from where you want to be.

162.

CAST AWAY JEALOUSY (KRIS)

Love is not jealous. Period. In fact, there is almost nothing that can suffocate a good feeling between two people faster than jealousy. It is, however, one of the easiest human emotions to understand. Jealousy stems from insecurity, and insecurity comes from feelings and thoughts of inadequacy.

There seem to be two essential ingredients that will help you cast jealousy out of your life. First and foremost, it's important to accept the fact that there is always going to be someone out there who has something you do not—more money, better looks, greater charisma, a longer list of achievements, or whatever. So what? Good for them. Stop comparing yourself to others and you'll be amazed at how much better you'll feel about yourself.

Second, in your relationships, try to embrace the idea that one person—whether friend, lover, or family member—will not fill all of your needs, nor will you fill all of theirs. And that's okay.

Most of us have witnessed firsthand how jealousy has smothered a relationship. When you find yourself feeling insecure or having feelings of inadequacy, try to gently reflect on your thoughts. See if you are busy comparing yourself to others. Are you making up stories that exist only in your mind?

163.

BE AWARE OF THE POTENTIALLY STRESSFUL EFFECTS OF YOUR PROMISES

It wasn't until a few years ago that I began to realize how often I made subtle promises to people during the course of a given day—and how often I regretted doing so.

Think about some of the promises we make to others that may not even seem like promises. Statements like, "I'll call you later today," "I'll stop by your office," or "I'll send you a copy of my book next week."

Let me be very clear about something. I'm not suggesting you stop making promises, or that many promises aren't necessary or important. Many are. What I'm suggesting is that a certain percentage of your promises (maybe even a small percentage) probably don't need to be made in the first place. And if they're not made, you will have less pressure to keep them!

I've learned to make slightly fewer unsolicited offers to do things for people. Rather than saying, "Hey, I'll send you a copy of that book we were discussing," I sometimes resist making the offer out loud. That way, I can still go ahead and send the book if I have time, but I'm not obligated.

With less on your plate, you can keep things in perspective and keep your priorities straight.

164.

CREATE YOUR OWN LUCK

Some people seem to get all the luck. Upon closer examination, however, you'd be shocked at the amount of "luck" that is self-created. The truth is, while luck is a factor of success from time to time, "lucky people" share some very consistent characteristics.

Lucky people are constantly putting themselves in the position to be lucky. They step up to the plate, they participate, they tell others that they are willing to accept help. I was "lucky" in a finance course I took at university many years ago. My friends couldn't believe the professor gave me an A for the course. What they didn't know was that I visited the professor and solicited his help *every single day* that he had office hours. The professor knew that I was trying hard and that I knew the material. Was I lucky? Sure, I was, but I had put myself in a position to be lucky.

Creating your own luck is sort of like planting a garden in an ideal environment. You'll be "luckier" with your plants if you provide the best soil, water, sunshine, and growing conditions. You might still get lucky and have a bumper crop without those things, but the odds are far less likely.

165.

STEP ASIDE FROM STUBBORNNESS

This past weekend one of my daughter's friends spent the weekend with us. Halfway through the weekend the two of them had a huge argument about some game they were playing. Their fun and laughter came to an abrupt halt. Because each of them was acting particularly stubborn, the argument ended up disrupting and interfering with a huge portion of their day.

I couldn't help but reflect on the destructive power of stubbornness; how being stubborn squelches our fun and interferes with the qualities of a nurturing and satisfying relationship.

Disagreements, failure to see eye to eye, and at least some conflict are inevitable. Looking back on our daughter's weekend, it's obvious that the problem wasn't really the argument, but the corresponding stubbornness. Had either girl simply said, "Oh, let's forget about it. I'm really sorry. Can we just start over?" there would have been a different outcome. The whole thing, regardless of what it was about, who started it, or whose fault it was, would have left like a passing storm, over in a matter of seconds.

It's the same with the rest of us. If we can drop our defenses, tame our ego, and let go of our need to be so stubborn, it's remarkable how quickly most issues will resolve themselves, painlessly and without too much effort. Success lies not in righteousness but in humility.

166.

EXAMINE YOUR RITUALS AND HABITS

When you work for a living, it's very easy to get into certain habits—some good, some not so good; some out of necessity, some by default. Many of these habits become so automatic that we never question, much less change, them.

Taking a close look at some of these habits and rituals, and being willing to change a few of them, can pay huge dividends in the quality of your life. Our habits are often enormous sources of stress in and of themselves.

Here are a few common habits, among hundreds of possibilities: You may be in the habit of not allowing yourself enough time to get ready before work and so are always in a hurry. You may be in the habit of eating a large lunch and always feel tired in the afternoon. Maybe you drink too much caffeine and feel nervous and agitated. Maybe you're a little grumpy in the morning instead of being friendly to your coworkers. Perhaps you go to bed too late in the evening. Only you know which habits are making your life more difficult.

Open your mind and imagine making a change! Everyone is different, and we all have different habits that get in the way of our happiness. What have you got to lose—except perhaps a little stress?

167.

UNDERSTAND SEPARATE REALITIES

If you have traveled to foreign countries, you're aware of vast differences among cultures. The principle of separate realities says that the differences among individuals is every bit as vast. Just as we wouldn't expect people of different cultures to see or do things as we would (in fact, we'd be disappointed if they did), this principle tells us that the individual differences in our ways of seeing the world prohibit this as well. It's not a matter of merely tolerating differences but of truly understanding and honoring the fact that it literally can't be any other way.

I have seen an understanding of this principle change lives. It can virtually eliminate quarrels. When we expect to see things differently, when we take it as a given that others will do things differently and react differently to the same stimuli, the compassion we have for ourselves and for others rises dramatically. The moment we expect otherwise, the potential for conflict exists.

I encourage you to consider deeply and respect the fact that we are all very different. When you do, the love you feel for others as well as the appreciation you have for your own uniqueness will increase.

168.

STAY FOCUSED IN THE NOW

Much has been written about the magical quality of "being in the moment." I believe, however, that this is one of those evergreen bits of wisdom that you can never quite get enough of. As you train your attention to be more focused in the moment, you'll be far less stressed out and hurried, more efficient, and easier to be with.

So often our attention wanders off into the future. We think (and worry) about many things all at once—deadlines and potential problems, what we're going to do this weekend, reactions to our work. We anticipate objections and hassles and things that are likely to go wrong. Or our attention is drawn to the past—we regret a mistake we made last week, or an argument we had this morning. We sometimes fret about "last quarter's poor earnings" or relive a painful or embarrassing event.

This quality of "being in the moment" has far more to do with what's going on in your mind than on what's going on around you. There will always be external distractions, the key element is how quickly you can bring your attention back to what you are doing.

There is something truly magical about getting completely absorbed in what you are doing. It increases your satisfaction immensely. I'm sure you're going to enjoy this one.

169.

DEVELOP YOUR OWN HELPING RITUALS

If you want your life to stand for peace and kindness, it's helpful to do kind, peaceful things. One of my favorite ways to do this is by developing my own helping rituals. These little acts of kindness are opportunities to be of service and reminders of how good it feels to be kind and helpful.

A helping ritual that I practice regularly with my two children is picking up litter in our surrounding area. We've become so accustomed to doing this that my daughters will often yell, "There's some litter, Daddy, stop the car!" And if we have time, we will often pull over and pick it up. We pick up litter in parks, on sidewalks, practically anywhere. Once I saw a complete stranger picking up litter close to where we live. He smiled at me and said, "I saw you doing it, and it seemed like a good idea."

Picking up litter is only one of an endless supply of possible helping rituals. Think of something that seems effortless yet helpful. It's fun, personally rewarding, and sets a good example. Everyone wins.

170.

RAISE YOUR STANDARD OF LIVING

Rest assured, I'm not referring to raising your material standard of living but rather the manner in which you live. One of my favorite quotes, from an unknown source, says it this way: "What you do speaks so loud that I can't hear what you say." Our lives really are our greatest message. The way we live—our integrity, honesty, humility, sense of well-being, compassion, generosity, willingness to forgive, and various other noble qualities—demonstrates, above all, the kind of person we really are.

The implications of raising the manner in which we live for our personal relationships is profound. As we raise our standards for ourselves, others will feel and may even be touched by the changes in our lives. In other words, as we become less selfish and greedy, others will be drawn to us. As we become kinder, softer, and perhaps a better listener, those whom we meet will relax around us and will want to share themselves with us.

There are many ways I'm trying to raise my own standard of living—I'm trying to become more patient, less inclined to interrupt others, and less hyper, to name just three.

There's no question that raising your standard of living—whatever that means for you—will reap huge dividends in the quality of your relationships. You'll see instant results with each positive change you implement.

171.

STOP COMMISERATING

Commiserating is a socially accepted form of complaining. We all do it, only to different degrees. Many people feel they are getting somewhere or getting some benefit when they habitually commiserate. Or they think "getting things off their chest" is a positive action. They associate the familiarity of commiseration with a feeling of relief.

Unfortunately, commiseration is a bad habit that only detracts from our lives. Our actions follow our energy, which includes our thinking and our conversations.

The next time you're at a social gathering, listen carefully to the ways people share their misery. Feel the energy of it all. Then, when you get home, sit quietly for a few minutes and consider what just happened. Try to tally up, in your mind, all the complaints. Now ask yourself: "What does it do? How far does it go toward solving problems, creating opportunity, expressing joy, and bringing forth creativity?" The answer is none, zero, zip.

Breaking this habit is difficult. It takes time, but it's worth it. The only way to quit is to notice yourself in the midst of commiseration or when you're about to commiserate. Gently remind yourself that, while it's tempting to join the others, you've got better things to do and dreams to pursue. As you avoid the tendency to commiserate, your rewards will be swift and certain.

172.

BE CAREFUL WHAT YOU ASK FOR

Many of us spend a great deal of time wishing things were different. Sometimes, the things we spend our energy longing for actually do (or would) improve the quality of our life. Other times, however, the very things we wish for are hardly worth the trade-offs or the effort.

The purpose of this strategy isn't to encourage you to stop dreaming of (or working toward) a better life, but to remind you that sometimes your life is pretty darn good exactly the way it is.

I've met plenty of people who spent years focused on how much better things would be when they were finally promoted to various positions—taking for granted the good parts of the job they already had.

A woman I knew worked hard to convince her boss that she could work remotely instead of coming into the office. She succeeded. The problem was, she never realized (until a month later) that, despite the dreaded traffic, she actually loved coming into the city each day. It was her social structure, her chance to be with people. After a while, she began to feel trapped in her own home.

The important point here isn't the specifics of the choice, but the recognition of the relevance of asking yourself the important questions—"What am I really asking for, and why?"

173.

EVERY DAY, TELL AT LEAST ONE PERSON SOMETHING YOU LIKE, ADMIRE, OR APPRECIATE ABOUT THEM

How often do you remember (or take the time) to tell people how much you like, admire, or appreciate them? For many people, it's not often enough. In fact, when I ask people how often they receive heartfelt compliments from others, I hear answers like, "I can't remember the last time I received a compliment," or "I never receive them."

There are many reasons why we don't compliment others. I've heard excuses like, "They don't need to hear me say that—they already know," and "I do admire her, but I'm too embarrassed to say anything." But when you ask the would-be recipient if he or she enjoys being given genuine compliments and positive feedback, the answer (nine times out of ten) is, "I love it."

Many people spend their entire lifetime wishing that other people would acknowledge them. They feel this especially about their parents, spouses, children, and friends. But even compliments from strangers feel good if they are genuine. Letting someone know how you feel about them is a gesture of loving-kindness. It means that your thoughts are geared toward what's right with someone. And when your thoughts are geared in a positive direction, your feelings are peaceful.

174.

ABSORB THE SPEED BUMPS OF YOUR DAY

Rather than labeling the issues that come up during a typical workday as problems, I think of them as speed bumps. Depending on how you approach and deal with the bump, it can be miserable or it can simply be a temporary slowdown—no big deal. If you step on the gas, speed up, and tighten the wheel, for example, you'll hit the bump hard! If, however, you approach the bump softly and wisely, you'll be over it in no time.

Problems can be looked at in a similar light. You can be annoyed by them, think about how unfair and awful they are, complain about them, and commiserate with others.

Thinking of problems as speed bumps encourages you to say things like, "I wonder what the best way to get through this one might be?" There is a healthy element of detachment involved, where you're looking at the problem objectively rather than reactively, looking for the path of least resistance. In other words, you assume there is an answer; you just need to find out what it is. This is in sharp contrast to seeing such concerns as problems, where it's tempting to think in terms of emergencies.

Problems can be really tough, but almost anyone can maneuver over a speed bump.

175.

SIT IN SILENCE

Without question, one of the simplest, most peaceful, and, I believe, most leveraged ways to maintain a loving connection is to practice the art of sitting together in silence. This beautiful yet seldom used practice brings forth compassion for one another while simultaneously strengthening the bond between you. Sitting with your partner in silence—or anyone else you have a close relationship with—can be powerful.

Think about the millions of words the average couple must share with one another over the course of their relationship: talking, arguing, negotiating, planning, remembering, bickering, and so forth. Few people, regardless of how many years they spend together, will set aside any time whatsoever to simply sit quietly together without saying a word. Yet this silent communication can be one of the most powerful and effective ways to communicate.

The practice itself is remarkably simple. You simply sit next to one another in a quiet, comfortable location. Close your eyes and clear your minds as well as you can. Breathe together, slowly and peacefully. Just sit, quietly and lovingly. Something magical happens when two people who share a connection sit together in silence. By the time you open your eyes, you'll feel more peaceful and loving—to one another as well as to yourselves.

176.

ARGUE FOR YOUR LIMITATIONS AND THEY'RE YOURS

Many people spend a great deal of energy arguing for their own limitations; "I can't do that," "I can't help it, I've always been that way," and thousands of other negative and self-defeating statements.

When we decide that something is true or beyond our reach, it's very difficult to pierce through this self-created hurdle. When we argue for our position, it's nearly impossible.

I had a client who told me, "I'll never have a good relationship. I always screw them up." Sure enough, she was right. Whenever she met someone, she would, without even knowing it, look for reasons for her new partner to leave her. If she were late for a date, she would tell him, "I'm always late." If they had a disagreement, she would say, "I'm always getting into arguments." Sooner or later, she would convince him that she wasn't worthy of his love.

She had to learn to stop expecting things to go wrong. She needed to catch herself in the act of arguing for her own limitations. When she started to say, "I always do that," she needed instead to say, "That's ridiculous. I don't always do anything." She had to see that arguing for her limitations was just a negative habit that could easily be replaced with a more positive habit.

177.

HAVE A CHOSEN CHARITY

Whether individually or through a business, there are so many good reasons to give to charity—need, satisfaction, compassion, desire to be of service, and more. If you run a business, having a specific organization you donate to is powerful. It gives your business a service-oriented focus and goal. Rather than some abstraction or last-minute tax planning, you know exactly—month to month—how much money your business is sharing. It's quite satisfying.

If you own your own business, this strategy is easy to implement. You just start doing it. If you work for a small business, you make your case to the owner. If you work for a large company, it can be trickier. In a large firm, there can be a silent assumption that "someone else will take care of it" or a feeling that no one would be willing to listen to your suggestion. But my guess is that most employers would love to contribute and probably already do in other ways. Many would welcome this suggestion. And if it doesn't work out, that's okay. You can implement a similar strategy in your personal life.

Someday, as you look back on your career, you'll probably be proud of many things. If you participate in giving to charity, this will be near the top of your list. Thank you for doing your part.

178.

BALANCE THE ACT (KRIS)

For most of us, life has become so crazy that it might be called a balancing act. Many of us are sped up, frenetic, nervous, and anxious about time. One of the keys to regaining a feeling of peace and composure is creating at least some degree of balance in your life. A nice way to think of balance is to see your life as a pendulum that swings back and forth. Its ideal location is dead center—perfectly balanced. When it swings too far to the left, you must make a few adjustments, enabling the pendulum to swing back to the right, and to find center again.

Years ago, Richard and I became aware of how out of balance and hurried our lives had become. It always seemed that we were running late, and we realized that we were trying to do too much. We had to let a few things fall by the wayside in order to come back to balance.

Choosing balance over chaos won't make your life perfect, but it will give you a much higher quality of life and deeper, more satisfying relationships. So, while we may never reach the perfect balance, any efforts we make in this regard will be well worth the effort.

179.

REMEMBER THAT EVERYTHING HAS GOD'S FINGERPRINTS ON IT

Rabbi Harold Kushner reminds us that everything that God has created is potentially holy. Our task as humans is to find that holiness in what appear to be unholy situations. It's easy to see God's beauty in a beautiful sunrise, the smile of a healthy child, or in ocean waves crashing on a sandy beach. But can we learn to find the holiness in seemingly ugly circumstances—difficult life lessons, a family tragedy, or a struggle for life?

When our life is filled with the desire to see the holiness in everyday things, something magical begins to happen. A feeling of peace emerges. When we remember that everything has God's fingerprints on it, that alone makes it special. If we remember this spiritual fact while we are dealing with a difficult person or struggling to pay our bills, it broadens our perspective. It helps us to remember that God also created the person you are dealing with or that, despite your struggle to pay your bills, you are truly blessed to have all that you do.

The fact that we can't see the beauty in something doesn't suggest that it's not there. Rather, it suggests that we are not looking carefully enough or with a broad enough perspective to see it.

180.

NEVER, EVER BACKSTAB

I was recently talking with a young man at a corporate function. He seemed nice enough until he launched into his backstabbing mode. Within ten minutes, I became an expert on the "dirt" in his company. The sad part of it was that this seemed to be a part of his ordinary conversation.

There are many reasons never again to backstab. First of all, it sounds terrible and makes you look really bad. When I hear someone slamming someone behind his back, it says nothing about the person they are referring to, but it does reflect poorly on the speaker.

Aside from being a mean-spirited and unfair thing to do, it's important to realize that backstabbing causes stress, anxiety, and guilty feelings in yourself.

Finally, it's absolutely predictable that if you backstab someone, you will lose the respect and trust of the people you are sharing with. It's inevitable that they will ask themselves the question, "If he will talk behind someone else's back, couldn't he do the same to me?" They know that the answer is yes.

No one bats a thousand. An occasional comment or the sharing of feelings probably isn't going to cause you great stress or ruin your reputation. But all things being equal, it's a really good idea to put backstabbing out to pasture, forever.

181.

RESIST THE URGE TO CRITICIZE

When we judge or criticize another person, it says nothing about that person; it merely says something about our own need to be critical.

Being critical not only solves nothing, it contributes to the anger and distrust in our world. After all, none of us likes to be criticized. Our reaction to criticism is usually to become defensive or withdrawn. A person who feels attacked is likely to do one of two things: they will either retreat in fear or shame, or they will attack or lash out in anger. How many times have you criticized someone and had them respond by saying, "Thank you so much for pointing out my flaws. I really appreciate it!"?

If, however, you take a moment to observe how you actually feel immediately after you criticize someone, you'll notice that you will feel a little deflated and ashamed, almost like you're the one who has been attacked. The reason this is true is that when we criticize, it's a statement to the world and to ourselves, "I have a need to be critical." This isn't something we are usually proud to admit.

The solution is to catch yourself in the act of being critical. Notice how often you do it and how bad it makes you feel.

182.

CONSPIRE TO INSPIRE

When you conspire to inspire, you do a lot more than act as a cheerleader for your partner or loved one's efforts. Your motivation is to help them become all that they can be—not necessarily what you want them to be, but rather you help them fulfill their own dreams and desires by believing in them, encouraging them, and sticking beside them in good times and bad. Even though you may not completely understand certain decisions they are making, you give them the benefit of the doubt, whenever possible. You seek first to understand and to be supportive.

When I was in college, I was a top-ranked tennis player. I knew, however, that I was ready to quit and change my trajectory. Virtually everyone gave me a difficult time, except Kris. She encouraged me in every way she knew to trust my instincts, follow my bliss, and "go for it."

It's never too late to start. All you have to do is make the decision to become a greater source of inspiration. If you're unclear about how to do this, ask your loved one! Ask the question, "What could I do—or how could I act—that would make me a greater source of support?" This may end up being one of the most important questions you ever ponder.

183.

ACCEPT THE FACT THAT, EVERY ONCE IN A WHILE, YOU'RE GOING TO HAVE A REALLY BAD DAY

Recently, I had one of those bad days that, in retrospect, was absolutely hilarious. It seemed that everything that could go wrong did. I was stuck in traffic on my way to the airport, spilled coffee on my shirt, my seat on the plane was given to someone else, I missed my connecting flight, a woman accidentally spilled her drink in my briefcase. After all of that travel hassle, I missed the two-thousand-person event I was traveling to because of a mix-up over entry access at the venue.

Disaster, right? Time to panic? Hardly. The way I look at it: Why should I be exempt from the rest of the human race? Let's face it. We all have really bad days every once in a while. It must have been my turn.

I've found that it's helpful to accept the fact that it's going to happen to you, too. This doesn't mean that you like it; only that you make peace with this inevitable fact of life. When you leave room in your heart for human error and tricks of nature, it allows you to keep your sense of humor, to not take yourself or your role too seriously, and to make the best of a bad situation.

184.

MASTER THE ART OF THE HEART-TO-HEART

Regardless of how good, honest, and loving your relationships happen to be it's inevitable that you are going to run into at least some degree of conflict. Every relationship has occasional issues to resolve. It's built into the system. That's why it's essential that you master the art of this type of communication.

A heart-to-heart is a very specific type of conversation that is ideally suited to—you guessed it—matters of the heart. You can use heart-to-heart talks to discuss awkward, painful, or difficult issues, or as a way to resolve conflict.

The foundation of a heart-to-heart talk is an agreement to approach the conversation with love and respect. Both parties agree to speak and, even more important, listen in a nondefensive manner to keep their hearts open and their reactions in check. The overriding goals of a heart-to-heart talk are to ensure that each person feels heard—and to ensure that both people emerge feeling closer to one another, regardless of any resolution.

This type of communication is easy to implement. In most cases, it only takes one person to positively influence the relationship by initiating this heart-felt communication. There's no formal structure to a heart-to-heart, nor is there a right or wrong way to do it. Be patient and, above all, loving.

185.

RECOGNIZE PATTERNS OF BEHAVIOR

No matter where you work or what you do, becoming an expert in recognizing patterns of behavior can help you reduce the stress in your life by eliminating many of your unnecessary interpersonal conflicts.

Most people (you and I included) have a tendency to repeat patterns and engage in habitual reactions. In other words, we tend to be bothered by the same things, irritated by the same sets of circumstances, and act defensively toward certain types of behavior.

Maybe a friend or coworker is someone who loves to gossip. By recognizing this pattern of behavior, you can avoid a great deal of potential grief. It doesn't matter whether you ask him not to—or that he promises that he won't—or that his intentions are pure. This doesn't mean he's a bad person, only that his pattern is that he can't help but gossip.

A person who is cheap today is almost always cheap. Someone who gets jealous usually does so on a consistent basis. Someone else who steals the glory does so whenever the opportunity presents itself.

By recognizing patterns of behavior, you are in the driver's seat at work. It helps you make the decision "not to go certain places" with certain people. Starting today, take a careful look at the patterns of behavior where you work.

186.

ASK YOURSELF, "WHERE IS THIS DECISION LIKELY TO LEAD?"

There is a story about "the trip to Abilene," and it goes like this: There were four friends sitting on a porch in a small town in Texas. It was a really hot day, well over a hundred degrees. Someone mentioned that there was a good restaurant over in Abilene, some two hundred miles away. Without knowing why, the four friends somehow ended up in the boiling hot car, headed toward Abilene. It was miserable.

When they finally arrived in Abilene hours later, one of the friends irritably asked, "Why are we here anyway?" It turned out no one had the slightest interest in being in Abilene. Everyone thought someone else really wanted to be there. No one thought to ask, "Where is this decision likely to lead?"

How many family get-togethers or business meetings are like this? Aren't there times when no one really wants to be there, but each person assumed that everyone else wanted to?

Many of us follow certain paths simply because they present themselves. Often, however, these paths lead you in directions or take you to places you really don't want to be. You can save yourself enormous amounts of time and energy by asking the simple, straightforward question: "Where is this decision likely to lead?" And then pay close attention to your answer.

187.

WRITE DOWN YOUR FIVE MOST STUBBORN POSITIONS AND SEE IF YOU CAN SOFTEN THEM

The first time I tried this strategy, I was so stubborn that I insisted that I wasn't stubborn!

Here are a few examples from my clients: "People who aren't stressed are lazy." "My way is the only way." "Men aren't good listeners." "Women spend too much money." "Children are too much work." "People in business don't care about anything except money." You can see that the list itself is potentially endless. The point here isn't the specifics of what you are stubborn about but rather the fact that you hold on so tightly to any given idea you might have.

It doesn't make you weak to soften your positions. In fact, it makes you stronger. I have a male client who was adamant, to the point of being obnoxious, that his wife spent too much money. As he relaxed a little and noticed his own rigidity, he discovered, to his embarrassment, that in reality he spent more discretionary money on himself than his wife spent on herself! His objectivity had become muddled by his own rigid belief.

As he has become wiser and gentler, his marriage has improved immensely. What are your most stubborn positions? Can you soften them?

188.

PAT YOURSELF ON THE BACK

At times, it's important to stop what you are doing and pat yourself on the back. Take a few moments to reflect on what you've been doing and on the nature of your intentions and actions. Mentally review your accomplishments. Think about how hard you work and how much you are contributing to your goals, and to the people you are working with.

As simple as this sounds, it really helps! I've done this many times, and have found that it puts things in perspective. Sometimes it reminds me of how busy I have become, which gives me compassion for everyone else who is busy. I can recognize why people sometimes forget or are unable to be appreciative—they are absorbed in their own work and their own lives.

Almost everyone loves to be patted on the back by others. However, when it's not happening, don't let it get you down or adversely affect your attitude. What you can do is praise yourself and pat yourself on the back. If you're doing a good job, say so. If you're making life a little better for even one person, or making any type of contribution to society, then the world is a better place because of you. You deserve to be recognized.

189.

SPEAK THEIR LANGUAGE

No two people are alike, and we all see the world through our own vision. We all filter information through a unique screen determined by our own personal history and the way we see the world. It's important to understand someone else's reality in order to effectively communicate with them.

I know a couple where the two partners are complete opposites. Joanne is highly intuitive and creative, and the epitome of a right-brain, emotional thinker. She can make instant, brilliant decisions based solely on her intuition and creativity. Ray is a type A, 100 percent left-brain, analytical thinker. To him, everything needs to make logical sense, or it's disregarded.

Their relationship greatly improved when each began to acknowledge their different styles of thinking and speak to each other in ways that felt most natural to their partner. Speaking to your partner or anyone else in "their" way all but ensures better communication.

We're all different in the ways that we think. Knowing this can give you the power to change the dynamics of your relationships, forever. Remember, your reality is not the reality—it's just yours. Start paying attention to people's communication styles and you'll be better equipped to meet them were they are.

190.

JUST FOR FUN, AGREE WITH CRITICISM DIRECTED TOWARD YOU (AND THEN WATCH IT GO AWAY)

So often we are immobilized by the slightest criticism. In truth, however, criticism is nothing more than an observation by another person about us, our actions, or the way we think about something, that doesn't match the vision we have of ourselves. Big deal!

When we react to criticism with a knee-jerk, defensive response, it hurts. We fill our minds with angry or hurtful thoughts directed at ourselves or at the person who is being critical. All this reaction takes an enormous amount of mental energy.

An incredibly useful exercise is to agree with criticism directed toward you. I'm not talking about turning into a doormat or ruining your self-esteem. But there are many times when simply agreeing with criticism defuses the situation, satisfies a person's need to express a point of view, offers you a chance to learn something about yourself, and provides you an opportunity to remain calm.

Give this strategy a try. I think you'll discover that agreeing with an occasional criticism has more value than it costs.

191.

LOWER YOUR EXPECTATIONS

I was sharing this idea at an event when someone in the back of the room raised his hand and said, "What kind of an optimist are you, suggesting that we lower our expectations?" His question was a valid one.

It's a delicate question to answer because, on one hand, you absolutely want to have high expectations and to expect that things will work out well. On the other hand, when you expect too much from life, when you are unrealistic and demanding, you set yourself up for disappointment and unnecessary grief.

Often, simply lowering your expectations, even slightly, can make your day (and your life) seem a whole lot easier. You can create an emotional environment for yourself whereby, when things do work out well, rather than taking them for granted, you'll be pleasantly surprised and grateful. And when your expectations don't go according to plan, it won't devastate you.

Many people confuse expectations with standards of excellence. Please understand that I'm not suggesting that you lower your standards or accept poor performance. Nor am I saying you shouldn't hold people accountable. What I'm referring to is making room in your heart for bad moods, mistakes, errors, and glitches.

So ease off your expectations a little, and see how much nicer your life can be. You won't be disappointed.

192.

STAY PLAYFUL

One of the most satisfying compliments I ever remember Kris and I, as a couple, receiving was from someone whom we have never even met. We were sitting in a movie theater waiting for the previews to begin. We were whispering, joking around, laughing, giggling, and just having a great time. I overheard the woman behind us whisper to her husband, "Look at those two, probably out on one of their first dates." At the time, we had been married for thirteen years!

When I think of all the people I have known over the years, a vast majority of the happy ones are, to one degree or another, playful. They can be serious in other ways, but in their relationships they have the capacity to be silly. When you're too serious, everything seems like a pretty big deal and it's easy to sweat the small stuff.

Many people make the mistake of telling themselves they will be playful "later," when all their business is taken care of and when all their problems are solved—but for now, they must be serious. The problem is, our "business" will never be completely taken care of, we will always have problems, and there's always something we must attend to. So, don't wait until it's too late—life is short; be playful now.

193.

PUT YOUR MIND IN NEUTRAL

One of the first observations I made when I learned to meditate was that my life seemed to calm down. Although I had the same responsibilities and identical problems, I felt as if I had more time, which made my work life become easier and more enjoyable.

While meditation isn't for everyone, there is a reasonable substitute that can be of tremendous help to anyone. It involves learning to put your mind in neutral, which you might think of as a form of "active meditation." In other words, unlike some forms of traditional meditation where you sit down, close your eyes, and focus on your breath, active meditation is something you can incorporate into your daily life.

Essentially, putting your mind in neutral means clearing your mind of focused thinking. Rather than actively thinking, your mind is in a more passive or relaxed state. When your mind is in neutral, your experience of thought is effortless yet completely responsive to whatever is happening in the moment.

When your mind is in neutral, thoughts seem to come to you as if out of the blue. New ideas and insights become a way of life because your mind, when it's relaxed, becomes open and receptive to your wisdom and unique greatness.

194.

SEARCH FOR THE GRAIN OF TRUTH IN OTHERS' OPINIONS

Almost everyone feels that their own opinions are good ones, otherwise they wouldn't be sharing them with you. One of the destructive things that many of us do, however, is compare someone else's opinion to our own. And when it doesn't fall in line with our belief, we either dismiss it or find fault with it. We feel smug, the other person feels diminished, and we learn nothing.

Almost every opinion has some merit if we are looking for it rather than looking for errors. The next time someone offers you an opinion, see if you can find a grain of truth in what the person is saying.

If you think about it, when you judge someone else or their opinion, it really doesn't say anything about the other person, but it says quite a bit about your need to be judgmental.

I still catch myself criticizing other points of view, but far less than I used to. All that changed was my intention to find the grain of truth in other positions. If you practice this simple strategy, you'll begin to understand those you interact with, others will be drawn to your accepting and loving energy, your learning curve will be enhanced, and, perhaps most important, you'll feel much better about yourself.

195.

ALLOW YOUR PARTNER A FEW ECCENTRICITIES

In a fun, innocent sort of way, our eccentricities help to define us. They outline our preferences and define us as unique and different from others. People have all sorts of eccentricities. Some people are a little obsessed with being clean. Others like to eat a certain food on a specific day, go to sleep at a certain time, or read at a certain time. There are endless examples.

One of the simple pleasures of life is feeling the freedom to be yourself and to do some things just the way you like to do them, without having to qualify your reasons or constantly explain yourself—as long as they aren't adversely affecting others. When you have the need to correct your loved ones, make them "wrong" or feel bad, or criticize their eccentricities, you rob them of a simple source of joy.

I'm not suggesting you buy into, encourage, or condone truly neurotic behavior—or anything that is disruptive or damaging. Instead, I'm referring to innocent little daily preferences that, for whatever reason, bring you (or your loved one) joy. I'm suggesting that when you allow others a few eccentricities, even if they conflict with the way you might do something, you'll be nourishing an important need of the human heart—the need to be oneself.

196.

BECOME LESS SELF-ABSORBED

To me, there are very few human qualities less appealing than someone who is highly self-absorbed. A person who falls into this category takes him- or herself extremely seriously. They love to listen to themselves speak and value their own time—but no one else's. They are usually quite selfish with their time, love, and money, in addition to lacking compassion for those less fortunate. Self-absorbed individuals see others and often treat others as instruments or objects to get something they want.

Don't confuse self-esteem with self-absorption. The two are completely unrelated. A person with high self-esteem loves others and feels good about herself. Because she already has what she needs in an emotional sense (feeling positive about herself), her natural instinct is to reach out to others in an unselfish way.

In contrast, people who are self-absorbed can be rude, insensitive to the feelings of others, and primarily interested in themselves—their own wants, needs, and desires. They tend to see people in a hierarchical manner.

It's a good idea to check in with yourself and make an honest assessment of your own level of self-absorption. Judge for yourself. If you feel you've drifted in that direction, then perhaps it's time to make a mental adjustment.

197.

DON'T RELY TOO MUCH ON DATA

It's often the case that when people get worried or frightened, they focus too much on data in an effort to alleviate their anxiety. The assumption is, "If I can figure everything out, everything will be okay." So worried stockbrokers will stare at their computer screens, gathering data instead of selling stock. Concerned homeowners will read thousands of reviews and never hire a contractor. All this data gathering may satisfy their curiosity and buy some time, but it will do little in a positive sense.

Of course, it's simple to justify our actions and decisions, especially when we're frightened. We can always rationalize that what we're doing is necessary and important. Sometimes this is true but not always.

A favorite quote of mine suggests that "If we had to overcome every possible objection before we got started, then nothing—absolutely nothing—would ever get accomplished." Excessive data gathering is very often the major factor that encourages us to overcome every possible objection before we get started, before we go out and do what it takes.

The next time you find yourself filling your head with facts and stewing over data, take a step back. It's very possible you have all the data you need and the simple decision to stop worrying is the most important thing you could be doing.

198.

THROW AWAY YOUR SCORECARD

If you wanted an absolutely predictable, completely reliable way to guarantee ongoing frustration—and a virtually guaranteed way to adversely affect your relationships and interactions—it would be to keep score of what you do, and of what other people aren't doing.

As ludicrous as this idea may seem, it's precisely what many people—partners, roommates, family members, and friends—do without knowing it, every day of their lives. This habit contributes to resentment, frustration, apathy, and an overall breakdown of an otherwise positive relationship.

When you engage in this extremely common habit, two things are certain. First, your excessive thinking about the perceived inequities in your relationship will frustrate you and stress you out.

Second, the other person will feel your resentment and built-up tension—which will give them more negativity to latch on to and think about.

As your scorecard enters your mind, see if you can drop those thoughts and bring yourself back to a loving feeling. It's easier to see your own contribution and to take someone else's efforts for granted. For the moment, reverse this thought process. Think not of what your loved one *isn't* doing, but instead think of what they *are* doing. You may discover that some portion of your frustration isn't reality, but simply a mental habit that has crept into your thinking.

199.

SEE THE GLASS AS ALREADY BROKEN (AND EVERYTHING ELSE TOO)

The essence of this Buddhist teaching is that all of life is in a constant state of change. Everything has a beginning and everything has an end. In our modern world, this means that every car, every machine, every piece of clothing is created and all will wear out and crumble. Our bodies are born and they will die. A glass is created and will eventually break.

There is peace to be found in this teaching. When you expect something to break, you're not surprised when it does. Instead of becoming immobilized when something is destroyed, you feel grateful for the time you have had.

The easiest place to start is with the simple things. Pull out your favorite drinking glass. Take a moment to look at and appreciate its beauty and all it does for you. Now, imagine that same glass shattered all over the floor. Try to maintain the perspective that, in time, everything disintegrates and returns to its initial form.

This philosophy is not a prescription for becoming passive or apathetic, but for making peace with the way things are. When your drinking glass does break, this philosophy allows you to maintain your perspective. Play with this awareness and you'll find yourself not only keeping your cool but appreciating life as never before.

200.

DON'T BE TRAPPED BY GOLDEN HANDCUFFS

The term *golden handcuffs* means that you voluntarily live at, or very close to, the edge of your current means (or, in many cases, well above). You trap yourself into keeping a job or career and working too many hours because that money is necessary to support your financial choices. The rewards of your income are overshadowed by the stress of maintaining your lifestyle. We get used to a certain lifestyle and can't imagine doing with less.

Obviously, this strategy doesn't apply to people who are living "on the edge," spending every dollar earned on actual necessities.

There is an effective way to deal with golden handcuffs. You can choose to lower your standard of living (that's right—lower), spend less money, consume less, and simplify your life. We all need to ask ourselves, "Are we really lowering our lifestyle if we are less stressed and worried? Would our standard of living be lessened if we created more time for ourselves and for the people we love? Are we really worse off if we are genuinely easing our financial pressures, and perhaps even carving out a little more time to enjoy our lives?"

So, take a careful look at your lifestyle and decide for yourself if this strategy is for you.

201.

UNDERSTAND THE STATEMENT, "WHEREVER YOU GO, THERE YOU ARE"

This is the title of a super book by Jon Kabat-Zinn. As the title suggests, wherever you go, you take yourself with you! The significance of this statement is that it can teach you to stop constantly wishing you were somewhere else. We tend to believe that if we were somewhere else—on vacation, with another partner, or in a different career—somehow we would be happier and more content. We wouldn't!

The truth is, if you have destructive mental habits—if you get annoyed and bothered easily, if you feel angry and frustrated often, or if you're constantly wishing things were different, these tendencies will follow you, wherever you go. And the reverse is also true. If you are a generally happy person who rarely gets annoyed and bothered, then you can move from place to place, from person to person, with very little negative impact.

Someone once asked me, "What are the people like in California?" I asked him, "What are the people like in your home state?" He replied, "Selfish and greedy." I told him that he would probably find the people in California to be selfish and greedy.

Something wonderful begins to happen with the simple realization that life, like a car, is driven from the inside.

202.

DON'T USE YOUR PARTNER AS A PUNCHING BAG!

Let's face it, most of us like to vent, at least once in a while. It just feels good to get certain things off your chest. And while venting is something I don't advocate as a therapeutic technique or as a way to relax, on occasion, I do it, too. For whatever reason, when you're frustrated, it sometimes feels good to share that frustration with someone you love. And even if it doesn't feel good, sometimes you just can't seem to help it.

There's an enormous difference, however, between an occasional venting session where you're letting off steam versus making venting an integral part of your regular communication. We've observed that in many relationships where one person is a regular "venter," the other person often reports feeling like a punching bag—the person who always receives the brunt of this wave of negative energy. This dynamic can appear in romantic partnerships, but also in friendships and with other family members.

Even though some venting is probably inevitable, there is a bit of selfishness involved as well. In other words, when we vent, someone else may be paying the price. So perhaps the best thing to do is simply be aware of how much venting is okay and how much is too much.

203.

GET REALLY COMFORTABLE WITH USING VOICE MEMO

The truth is, even the longest voice memo, if it's effective, is a huge time-saver and an excellent communication tool.

In a voice memo or voice note, you can leave very detailed, specific information and respond carefully and accurately to specific questions or concerns, all the while allowing the other person the luxury of reflecting on your comments, hearing them several times, if necessary, and listening at their leisure. Voice memos are an excellent way to explain a point of view with the luxury of being uninterrupted. It's also a great chance for someone to listen to a message without reactions such as defensiveness, or making a decision, or jumping to conclusions before hearing all the facts.

As writing partners, my dear friend Benjamin and I put together four entire anthologies using voice messages more than 90 percent of the time. Since both of us had full-time jobs, we were able to send thoughts and ideas during our breaks in the day. We've discussed the issue many times and both agree that had we chosen to communicate in person the bulk of the time rather than by voice memo, it's probable that none of the books would have ever been written.

204.

STOP BEING SO DEMANDING

Pause for a moment and reflect on how it feels when someone acts demanding toward you. What's it like when they are impatient, bossy, and picky? How does it feel when someone is looking over your shoulder making sure you're doing your part? The answer to these questions can be summarized in a single word: yuck!

Invariably, the person on the receiving end of the demands will ask herself the question, "What right does he have to treat me like that?" It's an excellent question.

It's easy to be demanding in subtle ways. We might, for example, demand to know where our partner is during every moment of the day. Or we might demand that the house look a certain way, and when it doesn't, we sulk or complain. Perhaps we demand that our friend or family members share certain beliefs or preferences.

Keep in mind that being around a demanding person is very stressful and no fun at all. It might be a good idea to consider the ways that you might be acting a little demanding. If and when you identify what they are, make a gentle effort to back off.

205.

BREATHE BEFORE YOU SPEAK

This simple strategy has had remarkable results for virtually everyone I know who has tried it. The almost immediate results include increased patience, added perspective, and, as a side benefit, more gratitude and respect from others.

The strategy itself is remarkably simple. It involves nothing more than pausing—breathing—after the person to whom you are speaking is finished. At first, the time gap between your voices may seem like an eternity—but in reality, it amounts to only a fraction of a second.

I spent most of my life waiting for my turn to speak. If you're at all like me, you'll be pleasantly amazed at the softer reactions and looks of surprise as you let others completely finish their thought before you begin yours. Often, you will be allowing someone to feel listened to for the very first time. You will sense a feeling of relief coming from the person to whom you are speaking—and a much calmer, less rushed feeling between the two of you. No need to worry that you won't get your turn to speak—you will. In fact, it will be more rewarding to speak because the person you are speaking to will pick up on your respect and patience and will begin to do the same.

206.

REALIZE THE POWER OF RAPPORT

The ability to establish rapport contributes to a more relaxed way of being. It helps you establish trusting, long-term relationships based on mutual honesty and integrity. In addition, the necessary ingredients of establishing rapport are identical to those that help you become a kinder, more patient, and relaxed person. So, you might think of establishing rapport as a form of self-therapy, a way to help you grow—personally, professionally, and spiritually.

When you lack a sense of rapport with someone, the problem can be difficult to describe. For whatever reason, you just don't click. Sometimes you can't quite put your finger on what's wrong—but something is missing.

The best way to establish rapport with someone is to assume that you don't have it. In other words, don't take for granted that simply because you know someone that your rapport is intact. Instead, take the time to reconnect. Be more interested in listening than in speaking. Be highly respectful and courteous. Demonstrate your sincerity and your genuine concern.

If you take the time and energy to establish rapport with others, your life will begin to change immediately. You'll have a better connection with people, which will create more nourishing interactions—personally and professionally. You will be trusted, loved, and admired, and you will become far more effective when dealing with others.

207.

ASK FOR "DREAM UPDATES"

Are you aware of your loved one's dreams—what they really want out of life? Are you sure? Or are you simply assuming that you know? Have you asked? If so, when was the last time?

It seems to us that many people have virtually no idea, beyond the superficial, of what their loved one's personal dreams really are. Sure, most people can say things like, "He wants financial security," or "She wants to be a mother." But beyond these almost universal preferences, an awareness—or sense of caring—for their dreams seems to stop.

There is something so rich and pleasurable about telling someone your vision, what you'd like to do, where you would like to go, and the contributions you'd like to make. And when the person you're sharing with is "right there with you," sharing your dreams, truly listening with interest and respect, your dreams come alive, and your shared experience can be almost magical.

The idea of asking for dream updates is a powerful strategy because whether or not the dream comes true is less relevant than the fact that your loved one knows and cares what you want.

So, starting today, make it a point to ask for a dream update.

208.

STOP WISHING YOU WERE SOMEWHERE ELSE

There are many ways that we spend time wishing we were somewhere else. We'll be at work and wish we were home. We wish we had different responsibilities or could spend our time with different people.

If you're not careful, you can begin to wish your life away, always wishing you were somewhere other than where you actually are. But you're not somewhere else. Rather, you're right here. This is reality.

But here's where this bit of wisdom gets a little tricky. When you're not getting any pleasure out of your situation, it's easy to say, "Of course I'd rather be somewhere else, I'm not enjoying myself." But step back and consider what's contributing to the lack of enjoyment. What comes first—a lack of enjoyment, or a mind that is focused elsewhere? Some of the time, the boredom or lack of satisfaction we feel is caused not by our careers or by how we are spending our time, but by the lack of focus in our thinking. The fact that you're thinking about where you'd rather be is literally sapping the joy out of what you're doing.

I think you'll be pleasantly surprised, even shocked, if you make the decision to spend less time wishing you were somewhere else and more time focused on what you're actually doing.

209.

BE GRATEFUL WHEN YOU'RE FEELING GOOD AND GRACEFUL WHEN YOU'RE FEELING BAD

The happiest person on earth isn't always happy. In fact, the happiest people *all* have their fair share of low moods, problems, disappointments, and heartache. Often, the difference between a person who is happy and someone who is unhappy is what they do with their low moods. How do they relate to their changing feelings?

Most people have it backward. When they are feeling down, they roll up their sleeves and get to work. They take their low moods very seriously and try to figure out and analyze what's wrong. They try to force themselves out of their low state, which compounds the problem.

When you observe peaceful, relaxed people, you find that when they are feeling good, they are very grateful. They understand that both positive and negative feelings come and go, and that there will come a time when they won't be feeling so good. To happy people, this is okay, it's the way of things. They accept the inevitability of passing feelings. Rather than fight their feelings and panic simply because they are feeling bad, they accept their feelings, knowing that this too shall pass.

Know that if you don't fight your negative feelings, if you are graceful, they will pass away just as surely as the sun sets in the evening.

210.

STOP SCRAMBLING

For many people, there are essentially only two speeds—fast and faster. It seems that, most of the time, we are scrambling around, moving very quickly, doing three or four things at once. Often, we are only paying partial attention or half listening to the people we are working with. Our minds are cluttered and overly busy.

In this hyper, frenetic state of mind, our concentration suffers. We waste precious energy and have a tendency to make mistakes. When we're scrambling, it's difficult to determine what's truly most relevant because we are so preoccupied with getting everything done.

As an experiment, see if you can make a conscious effort to slow down—both your thinking and your actions. You'll be pleasantly surprised to discover that, despite the slower speed, you'll become more relaxed and far more effective. The reason this happens is that you'll regain your composure and be able to see the bigger picture.

I operate at about half the speed I did ten years ago. However, I get about twice as much work accomplished! It's actually quite remarkable how much you can do when you're calm and collected. And more important, you enjoy what you are doing far more than when you're rushing around. It's often the case that you'll get more done in less time when you stop scrambling so much.

211.

ASK THE QUESTION, "WHOSE QUIRK IS THIS, ANYWAY?" (KRIS)

Isn't it usually the day-to-day, wash-the-toothpaste-down-the-sink kind of stuff about living with someone that can drive us crazy? It's funny, but you can love someone deeply and still be easily bothered by the simple act of sharing space with them. If the same things are bothering you over and over again, it helps to ask yourself the question, "Whose quirk is this, anyway?"

I heard the story of a couple, for example, where the wife (Pamela) is relatively clean, and the husband (David) is obsessively neat. One night, Pamela left a piece of lettuce in the sink after doing the dishes. David stood at the kitchen sink and yelled out at the top of his lungs, "Pamela, are you going to get over here and finish cleaning up your mess in the kitchen?"

Now, whose quirk is this, anyway? Obviously his.

When it comes to minor, everyday irritations, whether it's how your spouse loads the dishwasher or how your coworker words their e-mails, keep in mind that we all have our own little quirks. Often, if you just stop for a moment and reflect on the situation honestly and with a little humility, you'll see an obvious solution, or you'll see the situation differently.

212.

BECOME A LESS AGGRESSIVE DRIVER

Where do you get the most uptight? If you're like most people, driving in traffic is probably high on your list.

There are three excellent reasons for becoming a less aggressive driver. First, when you are aggressive, you put yourself and everyone around you in extreme danger. Second, driving aggressively is extremely stressful. Your blood pressure goes up, your grip on the wheel tightens, your eyes are strained, and your thoughts are spinning out of control. Finally, you end up saving no time in getting where you want to go.

Recently, I was driving south from Oakland to San Jose. Traffic was heavy but moving. I noticed an extremely aggressive and angry driver weaving in and out of the lanes, speeding up and slowing down. I continued on, listening to an audiobook and daydreaming along the way. As I was exiting the freeway, the aggressive driver came up behind me and raced on by. Without realizing it, I had actually arrived in San Jose ahead of him!

When you make the conscious decision to become a less aggressive driver, you begin using your time in the car to relax. Try to see your driving not only as a way of getting you somewhere but as a chance to breathe and to reflect.

213.

ASK YOURSELF THE QUESTION, "AM I MAKING THE ABSOLUTE BEST OF THIS MOMENT?"

If you were to make the most of this particular moment, and then do the same in all future moments, life would have a magical way of working itself out. You would be effective and productive and, most important, it would be very difficult for things to bug you.

Whenever you are feeling overwhelmed or stressed at work, ask yourself the question, "What am I doing with this moment?" Are you thinking about something stressful? Are you reinforcing a negative belief? Or are you using the present moment to its fullest advantage? Is your attitude and thinking pointed in a positive direction? Are you being solution-oriented?

I started practicing this strategy several years ago and have discovered something truly remarkable. It seems that in most instances when I'm feeling negative, overwhelmed, or pessimistic, I can improve my state of mind by checking in with this question.

When you're making the best of this moment, it's unlikely that you'll be sweating the small stuff because you'll be focused on solutions and enjoyment instead of problems and concerns.

214.

RELAX

What does it mean to relax? Despite hearing this term thousands of times during the course of our lives, very few people have deeply considered what it's really about.

When you ask people (which I have done many times) what it means to relax, most will answer in a way that suggests that relaxing is something you plan to do later—you do it on vacation, in a hammock, when you retire, or when you get everything done. This implies, of course, that most other times (the other 95 percent of your life) should be spent nervous, agitated, rushed, and frenzied. Most of us postpone relaxation until our inbox is empty. Of course it never is.

It's useful to think of relaxation as a quality of heart that you can access on a regular basis rather than something reserved for some later time. You can relax now. It's helpful to remember that relaxed people can still be superachievers and, in fact, that relaxation and creativity go hand in hand.

Being more relaxed involves training yourself to respond differently to the dramas of life—turning your melodrama into a mellow-drama. It comes, in part, from reminding yourself over and over again (with loving-kindness and patience) that you have a choice in how you respond to life.

215.

BECOME A WORLD-CLASS LISTENER

Becoming a world-class listener does two things. First, and most obviously, it nourishes your loved ones by demonstrating on a moment-to-moment basis that you truly care about what they have to say.

Secondly, effective listening greatly reduces your propensity to overreact to, or get upset by, little things. When you listen carefully and lovingly to someone, it will, in most cases, prevent you from jumping to conclusions or reacting habitually.

The only way to become an expert listener is the old-fashioned way—lots of practice. The good news is, anyone can become a better listener, simply by having the genuine desire to do so. All you have to do is observe how tempting it is to butt in, interrupt, or offer some feedback before the person with whom you're speaking is finished and before you understand what he is trying to say. You'll probably have to catch yourself many times before your habit is under control, but it will get easier with each passing day. As you nip this problem in the bud and as you become at least as interested in listening as you are in speaking, you'll be paving the way to a rare treat—a mutually respectful and satisfying interaction grounded in world-class listening. What could be better than that?

216.

RECOVER QUICKLY

There will be times when you make mistakes, sometimes big ones. There will be times when you overreact, offend someone, overlook the obvious, slip up, say something you shouldn't have, and so forth. The question isn't whether you will mess up, but rather how quickly you can recover when you do.

I remember an incident where I was taking credit for something that, in retrospect, didn't really belong to me. I was acting defensive and stubborn, and the person who felt slighted by me became angry and hurt. I was sharing my story with a friend who said, "Richard, it seems to me you were really stealing her glory." He explained his rationale, and I felt embarrassed and a little stupid. Later that day, I called the person to offer my sincere apology, which, to my relief, was accepted. All she really wanted was a simple acknowledgment for her actions and an apology from me. Had I done so earlier and recovered more quickly, a great deal of frustration and wasted energy could have been avoided.

If we're able to see our mistakes, admit to them, and move on, we can recover more quickly. Once you recognize the truth of the adage "To err is human, to forgive is divine," you create the emotional climate to recover from practically any mistake and move on.

217.

TURN YOUR MELODRAMA INTO A MELLOW-DRAMA

In a certain respect, this strategy is just another way of saying, "Don't sweat the small stuff." Many people live as if life were a melodrama—"an extravagantly theatrical play in which action and plot predominate." Sound familiar? In dramatic fashion, we blow things out of proportion and make a big deal out of little things.

I've found that simply reminding myself that life doesn't have to be a soap opera is a powerful method of calming down. When I get too worked up or start taking myself too seriously (which happens more than I like to admit), I say to myself something like, "Here I go again. My soap opera is starting." Almost always, this takes the edge off my seriousness and helps me laugh at myself. Often, this simple reminder enables me to change the channel to a more peaceful station. My melodrama is transformed into a "mellow-drama."

The next time you feel stressed out, experiment with this strategy—remind yourself that life isn't an emergency and turn your melodrama into a mellow-drama.

218.

DON'T LET YOUR OWN THOUGHTS STRESS YOU OUT

Think about how often we all have conversations in the privacy of our own minds. It happens, practically nonstop, all day long, every day of our lives.

When we are thinking, however, it's easy to lose sight of the fact that we think thoughts, not reality. It may seem strange, but most of us have a tendency to forget that we're thinking because it's something that we're always doing—like breathing. Thinking works in a similar way. Because it's such a part of us, we tend to give enormous significance and take very seriously most of the thoughts that drift through our minds. We begin to treat our thoughts as if they were the real thing, allowing them to stress us out.

When you have a thought, that's all it is—a thought. Thoughts certainly don't have the power or authority to stress you out without your conscious or unconscious consent.

The next time you find yourself having a "thought attack," see if you can catch yourself. Then say something gentle to yourself like, "Whoops, there I go again," as a way of reminding yourself that you're taking your own thoughts a little too seriously. I hope you'll take this strategy to heart—it will make a world of difference.

219.

DON'T SPEAK FOR YOUR SPOUSE (OR ANYONE ELSE!)

"I hate it when she speaks for me." "I can't stand it when he puts words in my mouth." I can't tell you how often I've heard these and similar statements. Just last week at a party, a man said to me, right in front of his wife, "She won't have any of those crackers. She doesn't like them." When he walked away a minute later, she said to me, "Would you mind handing me one of those crackers? I love them." When I hesitated for a split second, she said, "Oh, don't pay any attention to him. I hate it when he speaks for me—he does it all the time."

It was such a habit that she had learned to expect it.

It's quite disrespectful to speak for someone else. It implies that you don't think the person you're speaking for is qualified to speak for themselves—you know them better than they do. You know what they want, what they're thinking, and what their decisions are going to be. They couldn't possibly change their mind or think differently this time. These disrespectful assumptions—combined with the fact that it's one of the things most adults can't stand—make speaking for someone else an excellent candidate to put on your "Try never to do this again" list.

220.

ENCOURAGE COMPANY STRESS-BUSTERS

It's certainly not always true, but often it's the case that employers really do care about their people in the organization. It's also very often the case that the reason nothing is happening in the way of stress-reducing efforts is that no one is suggesting any changes.

Even if you can't persuade your employer to make any changes, it's often stress-reducing to hear their side of the story. The changes you'd like to see may be impossible, yet you might discover that there are people in your company—people just like you—who do care about your stress level and would like very much to do something about it.

Not all companies are open-minded, and you certainly wouldn't want to feel defeated if you can't pull it off, but it's almost always worth the effort to propose changes that would make employees feel less stressed.

Happy employees who don't feel overstressed are usually more productive, less adversarial, and more loyal. They are also less likely to quit or feel bitter toward their employer than those who feel stressed out and unappreciated. Sometimes if you can gently remind your employer of these facts, it really can make a difference. I hope it can happen for you.

221.

READ ARTICLES AND BOOKS WITH ENTIRELY DIFFERENT POINTS OF VIEW FROM YOUR OWN AND TRY TO LEARN SOMETHING

Have you ever noticed that practically everything you read justifies and reinforces your own opinions and views on life? We form opinions and then spend our entire lifetime validating what we believe to be true. This rigidity is sad because there is so much we can learn from points of view that are different from our own. A closed mind is always fighting to keep everything else at arm's length.

We forget that we're all equally convinced that our way of looking at the world is the only correct way. We forget that two people who disagree with one another can often use the identical examples to prove their own point of view—and both sides can be articulate and convincing.

Knowing this, we can either buckle down and get even more stubborn—or we can lighten up and try to learn something new! For just a few minutes a day—whatever your slant on life—try making a gentle effort to read articles and books with different points of view. You don't need to change your core beliefs or your deepest held positions. All you're doing is expanding your mind and opening your heart to new ideas.

222.

GIVE UP YOUR FEAR OF DISAPPROVAL

How many people choose careers and career directions based on what other people—parents, relatives, professors, friends—think they should do. "You should be a doctor, lawyer, pilot, musician" can be a very powerful message, especially when it's repeated often and associated with status, prestige, social approval, and other psychological accolades.

The message of this strategy is enormously important: our best chance of success is obtained through the elimination of fear. This includes the fear of disapproval from others. Examine the reasons behind some of your key life choices. Was it out of joy and genuine interest? Or was there an element of pleasing Mom and Dad, or someone else? Did you do it for the attention you thought you were going to get? If the answer to these questions is "yes," it might be time to investigate something new.

If necessary, talk to a therapist or counselor who might be able to shed some light on the subject or offer some helpful guidance. Whatever it takes, it's well worth the effort. If you change direction and do something because you truly love it, instead of because you think it's the "right thing to do," your path toward success might be closer than you ever dreamed possible.

223.

SEE BEYOND THE ROLES

It's almost inevitable that you will (at least on occasion) have a tendency to see people as their role instead of remembering the person behind the role. A baker has a life of her own, her own stories and dramas to deal with. The CEO is tired and can't wait to get home. Whether it's your staff or your boss, it's all the same. We're all in this together.

How often is our first question, "What do you do?" Or how often do we describe someone as "an accountant," or "a lawyer," as if the role were really who that person is? If we choose to, we can begin to shift the way we see and label others and in doing so make our life so much more pleasant.

When you see people as human beings first—their role second—the people you are in contact with sense your deeper perspective. You also open the door for much richer, nourishing, and more genuine interactions.

My suggestion is simply to remember that each person is special and so much more than what they do. Each person you meet has feelings—sadness, joy, fears, and all the rest. Simply knowing this and keeping it in mind can transform your life in some simple yet powerful ways.

224.

STOP REHEARSING UNHAPPINESS

Implementing this strategy can be a little tricky, but once you get the hang of it, it has the power to improve and even transform your relationships.

Here's an example: Kelly is driving to see her boyfriend. She remembers a fight from a few weeks ago, and she plays it out again, in her mind, almost as if it were happening right there. She begins to wonder if he's the right guy after all. Within a matter of minutes, she's a little angry, and by the time she arrives at his apartment, she's feeling slightly distant.

I refer to this type of inner dialogue as a "thought attack" because, in a sense, that's what it really is—your own thoughts attacking you. We get lost in our thoughts. We take out our self-created frustration on our loved ones as if they were the real problem. And while it's possible there is a real problem, our minds have a way of blowing things out of proportion.

The solution is simple but not easy. You have to catch yourself engaging in these tricky thought attacks. The idea is to see it happening while it's happening. You observe yourself as the thinker. Once you see it, the rest is easy. You simply drop the thoughts, dismiss them, and let them go.

225.

AVOID THE TENDENCY TO PUT A COST ON PERSONAL THINGS

I've known quite a number of people who rarely take days off to spend time relaxing or doing something just for fun because the "cost is too high." They make the mistake of calculating what they could be earning during the days, or even hours, they are away.

One of my fondest memories was when my dad took the day off to help me move. He was running a giant company at the time, and his time was extremely valuable. I remember thinking I was being clever when I said, "Dad, this is probably the costliest move ever made," since he could have easily hired movers to help me at a tiny fraction of the cost of his being there with me. Without even thinking about it, he looked at me and said, "Rich, you can't put a price tag on spending time with your son. There's nothing in the world I'd rather be doing than spending time with you."

Those words will stick with me for the rest of my life.

If you want to reduce the stress in your life and be a happier person, I have found it useful to look at certain issues without attaching a price to them—like spending time with someone you love.

226.

BE AWARE OF YOUR UNIQUE "STACKING ORDER"

The idea of a stacking order was introduced to me by a successful computer consultant. Essentially, the concept exists to help you clarify, in your own mind, how much work, or how many projects or tasks, you are comfortable working on at any given time.

We each have very unique temperaments regarding an optimal pace to work, how much we can handle, how much is "on our plate," at any given time.

Many people can relate to this concept in their personal reading habits. Some people love to read one book at a time. They enjoy each page and won't even think of picking up another until they are completely finished. Other people love to have five or six books going at once. They will read a chapter or two in one book, put it down, and perhaps not pick it up again for several weeks. If you forced people to ignore their reading preference (their stacking order), you would take them out of their natural rhythm and ruin their experience of reading.

The way we approach tasks, both personal and professional, is very similar, although most people never even consider it to be a factor. I hope you'll seriously consider your own stacking order. If you do, you'll discover a pace that's just right for your own temperament.

227.

DO ONE THING AT A TIME

The other day I was driving on the freeway and noticed a man who, while driving in the fast lane, was shaving, drinking a cup of coffee, and reading the newspaper! "Perfect," I thought to myself, as just that morning I was trying to think of an appropriate example to point out the craziness of our frenzied society.

When you do too many things at once, it's impossible to be present-moment oriented. Thus, you not only lose out on much of the potential enjoyment of what you are doing, but you also become far less focused and effective.

An interesting exercise is to block out periods of time where you commit to doing only one thing at a time. Whether you're washing dishes, talking on the phone, driving a car, playing with your child, talking to your spouse, or reading a magazine, try to focus only on that one thing. Be present in what you are doing. Concentrate. You'll notice two things beginning to happen. First, you'll actually enjoy what you are doing, even something mundane like washing dishes or cleaning out a closet. When you're focused, rather than distracted, it enables you to become absorbed and interested in your activity, whatever it might be. Second, you'll be amazed at how quickly and efficiently you'll get things done.

228.

COUNT TO TEN

When I was growing up, my father used to count out loud to ten when he was angry with my sisters and me. It was a strategy he, and many other parents, used to cool down before deciding what to do next.

I've improved this strategy by incorporating the use of the breath. All you have to do is this: When you feel yourself getting angry, take a long, deep inhalation, and as you do, say the number one to yourself. Then, relax your entire body as you breathe out. Repeat the same process with the number two, all the way through at least ten (if you're really angry, continue to twenty-five). What you are doing here is clearing your mind with a mini version of a meditation exercise. The combination of counting and breathing is so relaxing that it's almost impossible to remain angry once you are finished. The increased oxygen in your lungs and the time gap between the moment you became angry and the time you finish the exercise enables you to increase your perspective. The exercise is equally effective in working with stress or frustration. Whenever you feel a little off, give it a try.

The truth is, this exercise is a wonderful way to spend a minute or two, whether you're angry or not.

229.

AVOID THE WORDS "I LOVE YOU, BUT"

There's no question that three of the most beautiful words in any language are "I love you." However, you can virtually destroy the beauty of these wonderful words by simply adding the word *but* to the end of the phrase.

Years ago, Kris looked me in the eye and asked me, "Are you aware that you have qualified your love for me twice in the past five minutes?" At the time, I didn't even know what she meant. Specifically, I had told her, "I love you, BUT I want you to stop keeping me waiting," and "I love you, BUT it bothers me when you assume I'll want to do something when your friends are involved."

Kris wasn't saying she was above criticism, or that I wasn't free to discuss issues with her. She was asking me to separate my "I love yous" from any issues I was having with her.

We often use this kind of qualification with our partners, our friends, and our children. It turns a statement of affection into a manipulative and self-serving lecture. Try to avoid connecting your loving praise with the things that are bothering you. When you feel love for someone, tell them. Likewise, when something bothers you, share that, too. Just don't do it at the same time.

230.

GIVE UP YOUR FEAR OF SPEAKING TO GROUPS

I've heard that public speaking is the number one fear in America. It seems that speaking to groups is even more frightening to people than air travel, bankruptcy, even death!

A fear as big as this one doesn't exist in a vacuum. It doesn't show up only on those occasions when you are called on to speak in front of a group. Instead, the stress associated with speaking in front of others looms over you, perhaps very subtly, if there is any chance whatsoever that you will ever need to speak in front of people. Whether you may be required to give a presentation, a sales pitch, the results of a report or study, an all-out speech, or simply share an idea with others, the stress factor is the same—enormous—if you're scared.

The way to get over this fear is to put yourself in situations where you are required to speak to groups. You can start really small—even one or two others is a great place to start. There are classes you can take, coaches who can help you, books to read, and tapes to listen to. There are a variety of methods and strategies to look into. In the end, however, you'll have to take the first step and get in front of people.

231.

PRACTICE BEING IN THE "EYE OF THE STORM"

The eye of the storm is that one specific spot in the center of a twister, hurricane, or tornado that is calm, almost isolated from the frenzy of activity. Everything around the center is violent and turbulent, but the center remains peaceful. How nice it would be if we too could be calm and serene in the midst of chaos—in the eye of the storm.

Surprisingly enough, it's much easier that you might imagine to be in the eye of a "human storm." Suppose, for example, that you are going to a family gathering that is going to be chaotic. You can decide to use the experience as an opportunity to remain calm. You can practice breathing. You can practice listening. You can let others be right and enjoy the glory. The point is, you can do it if you set your mind to it.

By starting out with harmless scenarios like family gatherings, cocktail parties, and birthday parties for children, you can build a track record and enjoy some success. Once you have mastered harmless circumstances like these, you can practice on more difficult areas of life—dealing with conflict, hardship, or grief. Start slowly and keep practicing, and pretty soon you'll know how to live in the eye of the storm.

232.

KNOW WHEN TO BET, WHEN TO HOLD, AND WHEN TO FOLD

Many people fail to recognize just how important timing really is. There are times when the best possible course of action is to do nothing other than hold on, do essentially nothing, be patient. Other times, of course, it's important or at least appropriate to expand, to grow, to move forward. Other times we can save ourselves a great deal of energy and stress by simply being willing to take a loss now, to fold, rather than lose everything later.

It's amazing how often problems can be overcome and new opportunities can be realized by simply quieting down "the inner chatter" of our analytical thinking so that we'll know what action (if any) to take. This quieting of the mind allows us to get out of our own way so that we can know how to put the odds in our favor.

Wisdom is knowing when to do what. It's about being flexible and being willing to change, to flow. And while this may sound obvious, many people make the wrong choices simply because their mind is too busy. My suggestion here is to simply quiet down enough to consider the facts. Act from a place of wisdom rather than simply reacting out of habit.

233.

REMEMBER, NO ONE CAN READ YOUR MIND

It seems to us that one of the worst mistakes many of us make in our relationships is that, without even knowing it, we assume, at times, that our partner, friend, or family member can read our mind.

I was talking to a friend when he started to complain of his wife's inability to stay organized. Finally, I asked him, "Does Carol know how much this bugs you?" It turned out that she had no idea that it concerned him in the least!

It's important to recognize this problem and to nip it in the bud for several reasons. First, it creates a great deal of grief and inner turmoil for yourself. Second, it's not really fair to the other person. Here you are steaming mad about something, and you don't even give them the courtesy of telling them what's bugging you. You're demanding that they read your mind! What chance do they have?

Pick a time when neither of you is in a defensive mood. Then bring up the issue gently and respectfully and see what happens. If at all possible, avoid the self-destructive thought, "They should know what I want or need." You'll make it easier on yourself and on your relationships if you go ahead and let them know.

234.

AVOID COMMENTS THAT ARE LIKELY TO LEAD TO GOSSIP OR UNWANTED CHATTER

If you're like most people, there are times when you make innocent, fairly benign comments to others about a variety of things. You'll say things like, "Did you hear about John?" "Have you heard about so and so?" or "Did you know that?" Sometimes you initiate the conversation. Other times you keep a conversation going without realizing that you're doing so.

On the surface, this may not seem like a really big deal until you consider how much time and energy you spend engaged in conversations that may not be entirely relevant or may not be happening at an ideal time. Think about how often you feel stressed for time or energy.

If you take a careful look at how you actually spend your time, you may come to the same conclusion that there are many instances when you're engaged in unimportant conversations, when you honestly don't have the time or energy to be doing so.

Obviously there are many times when you want to be engaged in conversation, and that's perfectly fine and healthy. The trick is to be aware of when you are conversing out of habit rather than by choice. The slightest shift in your awareness in this tendency can pay tremendous dividends in the quality of your work life.

235.

FIND A MENTOR

I've never seen or even heard of someone moving backward as a result of finding a mentor. Yet when I ask around, very few people admit to having one.

I have had several mentors in my life who have helped me enormously in many aspects of life—business, money making, investments, marketing, public speaking, even physical fitness. Both the mentor and the student get a great deal out of the relationship, it's an ideal trade-off. The advantages to the student are obvious: confidence, camaraderie, ideas—a road map to follow. For the mentor, there's the joy of helping, feeling appreciated and needed, the fun of teaching, the privilege of reviewing what he or she did right over the years, the idea of passing the torch. It's a blessing to know that your ideas are being used by someone else.

Don't let anything stand in the way of finding an excellent, caring mentor. You will avoid many unnecessary mistakes and reap the rewards for years to come. Often, the best way to pay back your mentor is to promise him or her that, once you are in a position to do so, you'll do the same for someone else.

236.

SHARE AN INSIGHT

An extremely effective way to learn to stop sweating the small stuff is to share a meaningful experience with someone you love. You might share an insight you experienced regarding a certain way to make your life less stressful, or a new way to look at a problem or a frustration.

The reason this process is so powerful is that it helps you put more emphasis and attention on what's right with your relationships and with your life—what's working, what you're grateful about, and what's not bothering you—these and other factors that keep you from sweating the small stuff. It also brings to the surface ideas and tips on how each of you can become more relaxed and loving.

The nice thing about insights is that they tend to feed upon themselves, particularly when shared with a loved one. It makes you wonder what good things might be in store for the rest of us if we choose to share our insights with the ones we love.

237.

BE FLEXIBLE WITH CHANGES IN YOUR PLANS

Once I get something in my mind (a plan), it can be tricky to let go of it and go with the flow. I was taught, and to some degree it's certainly true, that success, or successfully completing a project, requires perseverance. At the same time, however, inflexibility creates an enormous amount of inner stress and is often irritating and insensitive to other people.

There are countless potential examples for all of us—times when our plans suddenly change, something we thought was going to take place doesn't, someone doesn't do what they said they would do. The question to ask yourself is, "What's really important?"

The more general question is, "What's more important, getting what I want and keeping my plans, or learning to go with the flow?" Clearly, to become a more peaceful person, you must prioritize being flexible over rigidity most of the time (obviously there will be exceptions).

You'll find that if you create the goal to become more flexible, some wonderful things will begin to happen. You'll feel more relaxed, yet you won't sacrifice any productivity. And the people around you will be more relaxed, too. They won't feel like they have to walk around on eggshells if, by some chance, your plans have to change.

238.

WHEN YOU SOLICIT ADVICE, CONSIDER TAKING IT

There are times when we share a concern simply because we want to vent or because we simply want someone to listen to us. But there are other times when we are genuinely confused about what to do and actively seek advice, such as when we say, "I wish I knew what to do," or "Do you have any ideas?" Yet when a friend, spouse, coworker, or someone else offers a suggestion, our immediate response is to tune it out or in some way dismiss it.

I don't know exactly why so many of us tend to dismiss the advice we receive. Perhaps we are embarrassed that we need help. Maybe we are too proud to admit that a friend or family member knows something we don't. Sometimes the advice we receive requires effort or a change.

The trick is to be willing to admit that other people can see things about us (or our circumstances) that we may be too close to or too personally involved with to see ourselves. So, while you probably won't want to accept all the advice that comes your way, you may want to become just a little more open to some of it.

239.

THINK OF WHAT YOU HAVE INSTEAD OF WHAT YOU WANT

In over a dozen years as a stress consultant, one of the most pervasive and destructive mental tendencies I've seen is that of focusing on what we want instead of what we have.

A friend of mine closed escrow on his new home on a Sunday. The very next time we saw him he was talking about his next house that was going to be even bigger! He isn't alone. Most of us do the very same thing. But happiness can't be found when we are yearning for new desires.

Luckily, there is a way to be happy. It involves changing the emphasis of our thinking from what we want to what we have. Rather than wishing your spouse were different, try thinking about her wonderful qualities. Instead of complaining about your salary, be grateful that you have a job.

Each time you notice yourself falling into the "I wish life were different" trap, back off and start over. Take a breath and remember all that you have to be grateful for.

Make a note to yourself to start thinking more about what you have than what you want. If you do, your life will start appearing much better than before.

240.

STAY AWAY FROM ULTIMATUMS

I once did a survey asking one hundred people if they liked it when they were given an ultimatum. Ninety-five people said no. The other five said some variation of "You must be kidding." I've never met anyone who likes ultimatums. Yet many people use this form of manipulation on a regular basis to get what they want. My experience is that, in one way or another, it almost always backfires.

There may be situations when you have virtually no option but to give someone an ultimatum—for example, "You must show up to work on time or you're going to lose your job." That's a different issue. But in personal relationships, ultimatums are rarely well received.

Not always, but often, an ultimatum stems from the fear that, in the absence of the ultimatum, you're not going to get what you want. So, out of desperation, you demand it, attaching a serious consequence—hoping that will do the trick. The problem is, you push the person away far more often than you frighten someone into doing it your way. So, stop giving ultimatums—or else!

241.

ACCEPT THE FACT THAT THERE'S ALMOST ALWAYS GOING TO BE SOMEONE MAD AT YOU

This is a difficult concept to accept, particularly if, like me, you are a "people pleaser." Yet I've found that if you don't make peace with this virtual inevitability, it guarantees that you will spend a great deal of time struggling with one of the unfortunate realities of life—disappointment.

The fact that someone is virtually always going to be mad or at least disappointed in you is inevitable because while you're busy trying to please one person, you're often disappointing someone else. If two or more people want, need, or expect something from you—and you can't do it all—someone is going to be left disappointed.

Your boss or client needs you to do something—the only problem is, your child or spouse needs you too at the same time. You're a waitress at a busy restaurant and every table seems anxious—you're doing the very best you can, but customers are still mad. You forget someone's birthday. Even though you remembered nineteen other birthdays, you still managed to upset one person. And so it goes.

When you make peace with this fact of life, a huge weight is lifted off your shoulders. You'll understand that there's simply nothing you can do—other than your best.

242.

CHANGE WHAT YOU CAN, ACCEPT THE THINGS YOU CAN'T

This strategy is adopted from the serenity prayer that says: "Lord, grant me the serenity to accept the things I cannot change, the courage to change the things I can, and the wisdom to know the difference." What an incredibly powerful message!

There are things we *must* deal with. There are things we can change, that we have some power to control. There are other things that are absolutely beyond our control. Yet how often do we spend our time and energy doing absolutely nothing about the things we do have some control over while complaining about those things we can't do anything about?

A friend of mine in real estate insists that many of his competitors failed, in part, because instead of focusing on what they could control, they spent their time complaining about bureaucracy and trying to get around the rules and regulations. In his words, "Dealing with bureaucracy is a part of the business." Learning to dance with the "what is" part of business—or life—instead of struggling against it can transform your approach.

Do something positive, something you have control over. Once you start thinking in these terms, you'll be amazed at how easy and enjoyable it is to create the abundance you desire and deserve.

243.

PRACTICE IGNORING YOUR NEGATIVE THOUGHTS

It has been estimated that the average human being has around 50,000 thoughts per day. Some of these thoughts are going to be positive and productive. Unfortunately, however, many of them are also going to be negative—angry, fearful, pessimistic, worrisome. The important question in terms of becoming more peaceful is what you choose to do with the ones that you have.

You can analyze your thoughts—ponder, think through, study, think some more—or you can learn to ignore them—dismiss, pay less attention to, not take so seriously. This latter option is infinitely more effective in terms of learning to be more peaceful.

When you have a thought—any thought—that's all it is, a thought! It can't hurt you without your consent. For example, if you think, "I'm upset because my parents didn't do a very good job," you can get into it, which will create inner turmoil. Or you can choose to dismiss the thought. This doesn't mean your childhood wasn't difficult, but in this present moment, you have a choice of which thoughts to pay attention to.

If you ignore or dismiss a negative thought that fills your mind, a more peaceful feeling is only a moment away. And, in a more peaceful state of mind, your wisdom and common sense will tell you what to do.

244.

TAKE ADVANTAGE OF YOUR COMMUTE

I was talking to an executive of a fairly large corporation who was complaining to me about his "nasty commute," which took almost an hour and a half each way. "Wow," I said, "that's too bad, but at least you're able to read some good books." His response shocked me. He said in a dead serious tone, "What are you talking about? I don't have any time to read." At first I thought he was kidding. Once I realized he wasn't, I said, "You mean you don't listen to audio books while you're in the car?" He shook his head no. "What do you do for those three hours each day?" He didn't seem to really know.

Assuming he works fifty weeks a year, he spends 750 hours a year driving to and from work. That's a staggering amount of time for anyone to waste, especially when there is such a great alternative.

You can see how incredibly valuable your driving commute time can be, should you decide to look at it that way. I love audio books. Try podcasts, audio books, listening to a meditation, audio-based language learning programs, or any other creative ways to take advantage of that commute.

245.

PREDICT THE PREDICTABLE

To one degree or another, all of us have a certain amount of predictability. Happily, learning to predict the predictable—and making peace with it—can save you from a great deal of agitation.

Kris was raised in Portland, Oregon, where it rains a significant portion of the time. You might prefer to bask in a little more sunshine, but in Oregon you certainly wouldn't complain, "I can't believe it's raining—my day is ruined."

You can extend this simple wisdom to your relationships. I used to get frustrated when Kris was running even a little late. After a while, however, I learned that it was part of her nature. But once it became predictable—and I accepted it—it became a nonissue.

All of us have habits, quirks, and reactions that are fairly predictable. When you let them go—instead of hassling your loved ones about them—you may be surprised at how often the issues fade away on their own. People change and grow, usually without our involvement. Over the years, for example, Kris has become far more punctual. In fact, today I probably run late more often than she does. It's a good thing I didn't give her too hard a time—maybe she'll be easy on me, too.

246.

THINK BIG!

The implications of thinking big are widespread and impressive. Thinking big is a magic door opener that broadens your perspective and allows you to see new opportunities. Thinking big makes life easier and a lot more fun.

As usual, the primary reason many people think too small is fear. Thoughts like "I can't speak to a room full of people," "I can't risk taking on a larger project," and "I couldn't ask the boss to have lunch with me" fill the mind and are taken too seriously. When fearful thoughts enter the mind, try to banish them. You can do it—once you believe you can. The fear you are experiencing is almost always self-created and usually unnecessary.

I have a friend who spent most of his adult life insisting he couldn't write a book. This was very puzzling to me, because not only was he an excellent writer, but he also felt quite comfortable writing articles and chapters! One day I asked him to consider the idea that a book is nothing more than a series of interesting chapters put into sequence. He had never thought of it in those terms. Instead, he had always focused on his stubborn belief that writing a book was too big a project. Two years later, he finished his first book.

247.

BE WILLING TO LEARN FROM FRIENDS AND FAMILY

One of the saddest observations I've made centers around how reluctant many of us are to learn from the people closest to us—our parents, spouse, children, and friends. Rather than being open to learning, we close ourselves off out of embarrassment, fear, or pride. It's almost as if we say to ourselves, "I have already learned all that I can [or want to learn] from this person; there is nothing else I can [or need to] learn."

It's sad, because often the people closest to us know us the best. They are sometimes able to see ways in which we are acting in a self-defeating manner and can offer very simple solutions. If we are too proud or stubborn to learn, we lose out on some wonderful, simple ways to improve our lives.

I have tried to remain open to the suggestions of my friends and family. In fact, I have gone so far as to ask certain members of my family and a few of my friends, "What are some of my blind spots?" Not only does this make the person you are asking feel wanted and special, but you end up getting some terrific advice.

248.

LET GO OF BATTLES THAT CANNOT BE WON

One of the major contributing factors to self-created stress is the tendency that most of us have to hold on to battles that we have virtually no chance of winning. We bump up against stone walls, but instead of backing off and taking the path of least resistance, we keep right on struggling.

Perhaps you're frustrated by the complaining of a coworker. For every valuable insight you share with her, she comes back with yet another, "Yeah, but..." and never, ever takes your advice. If you're frustrated by this type of typical interaction, it's because you're fighting a battle that can't be won. She's probably going to be complaining for the rest of her life.

Does this mean you should stop caring? Of course not. It simply means you can dismiss the idea that you are ever going to convince her to stop complaining. Case closed.

Obviously, if something legitimate or terribly important is at stake, you may have to prove your position and it will be worth the trouble. Most of the time, however, that's not where daily frustration stems from. In fact, most of us handle the "big stuff" pretty well. The stress you feel often comes from fighting those "no chance of winning" battles where the outcome is practically irrelevant anyway.

249.

BE HAPPY WHERE YOU ARE

Sadly, many of us continually postpone our happiness—indefinitely. We keep convincing ourselves, "Someday I'll be happy." We convince ourselves that life will be better after we get married, have a baby, then another. Then we are frustrated that the kids aren't old enough—we'll be more content when they are. After that, we're frustrated that we have teenagers to deal with. We tell ourselves that our life will be complete when our spouse gets his or her act together, when we get a nicer car, are able to go on a nice vacation, when we retire. And on and on and on!

Meanwhile, life keeps moving forward. The truth is, there's no better time to be happy than right now. If not now, when? One of my favorite quotes comes from Alfred D'Souza. He said, "For a long time it had seemed to me that life was about to begin—real life. But there was always some obstacle in the way, something to be got through first, some unfinished business, time still to be served, a debt to be paid. Then life would begin. At last it dawned on me that these obstacles were my life." This perspective has helped me to see that there is no way to happiness. Happiness is the way.

250.

DON'T FIGHT UNLESS THE MOOD IS RIGHT

Moods are really funny things. On one hand, when your mood is up and you're feeling good, life looks pretty darn good. Generally speaking, your relationships look pretty good, too. You feel secure, loving, and satisfied. You find it easy to compromise and forgive.

On the other hand, when your mood is down and you're feeling grumpy, agitated, and stressed, your life looks drastically different—particularly your relationships. All of a sudden, you're feeling dissatisfied, as if something were missing.

But there's hope! Despite their apparent power, the effect of moods on your relationship can be minimized. All that is required is a respect for the illusion of moods along with the willingness to make certain allowances for your moods—and the moods of others—when they occur. Your moods are going to continue to come and go as they always have, but you can learn to respond to them in an entirely new way.

Your awareness of the deceptive nature of low moods can eliminate a great deal of frustration—and will most certainly keep you from blowing many things out of proportion. Reactivity will be replaced by compassion. So, go ahead and fight—but wait until the mood is right.

251.

THINK OF STRESS AND FRUSTRATION AS DISTRACTIONS TO YOUR SUCCESS

Many people assume that stress and success are linked in the same way that glue sticks to paper. The assumption is, "There's a huge price to pay in order to achieve your dreams, and stress is an inevitable and essential part of the process." People think of their stress as a source of motivation. Thus, they begin to look and behave in very stressful ways—they become short-tempered and poor listeners. They lose their perspective and wisdom. In short, they sweat the small stuff—big time!

The problem is, if you assume that stress is a positive and necessary factor, you're going to create—knowingly or unknowingly—a great deal more of it. If, however, you can begin to think of stress as a distraction, you can begin to rid yourself of a great deal of it.

Stress is, in fact, a distraction. It interferes with clear and logical thinking. It makes wisdom, insights, and creativity more difficult to bring forth. Stress is also exhausting, robbing you of valuable and precious energy—both physical and emotional.

My suggestion is this: when you begin sweating the small stuff at work, gently remind yourself that, while work may be difficult, the stressful feelings you are experiencing aren't helping and certainly aren't worth defending.

252.

REMEMBER, YOU BECOME WHAT YOU PRACTICE MOST

Repeated practice is one of the most basic principles of most spiritual and meditative paths. In other words, whatever you practice most is what you will become. If you are in the habit of being uptight whenever life isn't quite right, reacting negatively to criticism, insisting on being right, allowing your thinking to snowball in response to adversity, or acting like life is an emergency, then your life will be a reflection of this type of practice. You will be frustrated because, in a sense, you have practiced being frustrated.

Likewise, however, you can choose to bring forth in yourself qualities of compassion, patience, kindness, humility, and peace—again, through what you practice.

This isn't to suggest that you make your entire life into a great big project where the goal is to be constantly improving yourself. Only that it's immensely helpful to become conscious of your own habits, both internal and external. Where is your attention? How do you spend your time? Are you cultivating habits that are helpful to your stated goals? Is what you say you want your life to stand for consistent with what your life really stands for?

If you remember that what you practice you will become, you may begin choosing different types of practice.

253.

DEVELOP RELATIONSHIPS WITH PEOPLE BEFORE YOU NEED SOMETHING

So many of us wait until we desperately need something from someone before we take the time to get to know them. In truth, this is probably the absolute worst time to do so. How much easier it is to work with people when they already know and trust you, when you know the names of their spouse and children, when they know that you care about their happiness and that you are a sincere, trustworthy person.

I make it a point to get to know as many people as possible in my own community. I'm friendly with the banker, the owners of the restaurants and coffee shops, the local mechanic, the pharmacist, the florist, and so many others. The result is that, if one of my children is sick, the local pharmacist will gladly take the time to discuss the issue with me. He's genuinely concerned about my family as I am about his.

This has nothing to do with taking advantage of people. It's just the way life works. People love to help those they know and trust. Each of these people, and so many others, know that I'll do (and have done) special things for them as well. In fact, I wouldn't think twice about it.

Instead of waiting until you need help, why not show people kindness right now?

254.

MAKE ALLOWANCES FOR INCOMPETENCE

Like so many things, incompetence can be represented on a bell-shaped curve. There is always going to be a small percentage of people who are near the extremes—outstandingly good and outstandingly bad—but most people will fall somewhere near the middle. In most professions, it's just the way life seems to pan out.

It's interesting, however, that so many people don't seem to understand this dynamic or, if they do, they certainly don't exhibit any compassion or common sense in their reaction to it. I've seen people so upset about obvious incompetence that I thought they might have a heart attack or a nervous breakdown.

In no way am I saying it's pleasant to deal with incompetence, but if you want to avoid feeling so irritated, it's important that you stop being so surprised and caught off guard by it. The next time you run into incompetence, even if it's flagrant, see if you can make the best of it, rectify the situation if possible, and then go on with your day. Let it go. Rather than turning the incompetence into front-page news in your mind, see if you can turn it into just another minor story. If you do, you'll be free from yet another of life's sources of frustration.

255.

KNOW YOUR OWN VALUE

Ideally, everyone who is in a friendship, partnership, or family would treat their loved ones as a 100 percent equal in every sense of the word. Unfortunately, however, we don't live in an ideal world. For a variety of reasons, there are some people who feel a sense of superiority. In some cases, they feel their role or contribution is more significant or important—especially in romantic relationships. In other cases, there is simple ignorance. Then there are those who have an unhealthy dose of arrogance or self-importance.

One of the greatest gifts you can give yourself and, ultimately, your relationships is to know your own value, to feel secure that you are special, unique, and important. There isn't a person in this world who is just like you, and no one could take your place. Your contribution is important, and the gifts and value you bring to your relationship are significant and irreplaceable.

Take time on a regular basis to remind yourself how special and wonderful you really are. If you do, you'll always know your own value.

256.

AVOID "IF ONLY, THEN" THINKING

Just as it sounds, "if only, then" thinking refers to the oh-so-common tendency to fill your head with thoughts designed to convince yourself that "if only" certain conditions were met—then you'd be happy. Here are a few examples: "If only I made more money, then I'd feel secure," "If only I received more attention or credit, then I'd feel good," "If only he (or she) were different, I'd have a better life." You get the picture.

In order to see the flaw in "if only, then" thinking, all you need to do is think back to a few of the thousands of times you told yourself essentially the same thing, and ended up getting exactly what you wanted, and you still weren't satisfied. Or if you were, it didn't last for long.

Obviously, I'm not suggesting that you don't have to know where you're going or that it's not important to have a plan and work hard. What I'm talking about here is the tendency to discredit or underappreciate the life you have now at the expense of some imagined future.

My advice is simple. Go ahead and dream your dreams and have a plan. But never forget that the secret to satisfaction isn't getting to some imagined destination, but in enjoying the ride along the way.

257.

QUIET THE MIND

Although there are many techniques for quieting the mind, the most universally accepted and regularly used technique is meditation. In as little as five to ten minutes a day, you can train your mind to be still and quiet. This stillness can be incorporated into your daily life, making you less reactive and irritable, and giving you greater perspective to see things as small stuff rather than as emergencies.

Meditation essentially involves emptying your mind. You close your eyes and focus your attention on your breath—in and out, in and out. As thoughts enter your mind, you gently let them go and bring your attention back to your breath. Do this over and over again. Over time, you'll train yourself to keep your attention on your breath as you gently dismiss any stray thoughts.

You'll quickly discover that meditation isn't easy. You will notice that your mind will fill with thoughts the moment you attempt to keep it still. It's rare for a beginner to be able to focus attention for more than a few seconds. The trick to becoming an effective meditator is to be gentle on yourself and to be consistent. A few minutes each day will reap tremendous benefits over time.

258.

DON'T BE TOO QUICK TO COMMENT

Many of us are quick to comment on practically anything. We'll gladly comment on someone else's comment, their opinion, or a mistake that we perceive may have been made. We will offer our own opinion, comment on a policy, a pattern of behavior, or a personal gripe.

Obviously, there are times when other people ask that we comment or share our point of view. And a great deal of the time we are simply being responsive to the moment, and our comments are absolutely appropriate. In fact, this is probably the case a vast majority of the time. Most of our comments are probably useful, helpful, or simply entertaining. Terrific. Keep commenting.

Invariably, however, some of our comments are at best unnecessary and at worst counterproductive. They arise out of habit, a knee-jerk reaction, or some unexplained need we have to comment. Some of these comments lead to arguments, hurt feelings, or confusion. These are the ones that you want to avoid making, if possible.

The question is: How much stress could you avoid by simply learning to bite your tongue when it's in your best interest to do so? I've met more than a few people who claim that this simple change in habit has greatly contributed to a more peaceful life.

259.

TREASURE YOUR LOVED ONES

One of the most life-affirming, love-enriching messages you can send to your loved ones is the message, "I treasure you." When someone knows they are treasured, they feel important and valued. This encourages them to treasure you back, to remain loyal and loving, and to feel as though your relationship is satisfying. When you get right down to it, letting someone know they are treasured is one of the greatest compliments you can give.

I have a close friend who is a psychologist specializing in marriage counseling. She tells us it's very common for people to know what their partner doesn't like about them—but to have no idea of what they like or appreciate. According to our friend, however, the slightest acknowledgment, and more focus on the positive, can turn a relationship around.

The best way to let someone know you treasure them is, you guessed it, to tell them. Let your partner, friends, children, or family members know, frequently, what you like about them. Be specific. If you like their smile, their laugh, something they do, whatever, let them know. Don't make the mistake of assuming that they already know what you like—they may not. You may not have told them for a long, long time.

260.

LET GO OF PERSONALITY CLASHES

The assumption is often made that certain personality types just don't mix—shy people can't get along with outgoing people, or sensitive individuals can't work well with more aggressive people, to name just a few. This is unfortunate because rarely can we pick and choose the types of personalities around us.

Like everyone else, I prefer to work with certain types of people over others. I've found, however, that with some gentle effort on my part, I can usually work well with practically anyone, regardless of their personality type. The trick, I believe, lies in the word *gentle.*

What works well for me is to think in terms of getting along as part of my job description. I attempt to take responsibility for making the relationship work; I put the ball in my own court. Instead of seeing myself as good and the other person as flawed, I humorously label each of us as "characters," each playing a different role. I keep my spirit light and my sense of humor intact. Almost without fail, this opens my heart and broadens my perspective.

Letting go of personality clashes in this way has made an enormous difference in my work life. I suggest you take a similar look at your own personality clashes. Letting them go will take a huge weight off your shoulders.

261.

TAKE UP YOGA

For centuries, yoga has been used to clear and free the mind, giving people feelings of ease and equanimity. It's easy to do and takes only a few minutes a day. What's more, people of virtually any age and fitness level can participate.

Although yoga is physical in nature, its benefits are both physical and emotional. On the physical side, yoga strengthens the muscles and the spine, creating flexibility and ease of motion. On the emotional side, yoga is a tremendous stress reducer. It balances the body-mind-spirit connection, giving you a feeling of ease and peace.

The effects of yoga are truly amazing. After only a few minutes, you feel more alive and open, peaceful and relaxed. Your mind is clear. The rest of your day is easier and more focused. I used to believe that I was too busy to practice yoga. I felt I didn't have time. I'm now certain that the opposite is true—I don't have time not to practice yoga. It's too important not to do.

262.

AVOID CORRECTING

I was in the lobby of a health club when a woman said to her husband, "See you later, honey. I've got to get home because I'd like to make you and the kids that dish you love so much. It takes over an hour and I want to have plenty of time." My heart sank when I heard her husband fire back, "No it doesn't—it only takes about fifty minutes." Ouch.

This is a somewhat obnoxious example of the tendency many of us have to correct one another, particularly those we are closest to. Yet it demonstrates how disrespectful and potentially damaging this habit can be.

Often, the "correction" is absolutely unnecessary. Other than being ignorant to the hurtful effects the correction has on the recipient, and the way it takes the joy out of sharing, the only possible motivation could be an attempt to be outright mean.

The lesson here is simple. No one appreciates being corrected. In fact, most people resent it. So, unless there's a really good reason or you're dealing with an extremely important issue, it's a good rule of thumb to keep your corrections to yourself. Your loved ones will be able to share with you freely and openly.

263.

MAKE SERVICE AN INTEGRAL PART OF YOUR LIFE

Several teachers and philosophers that I have learned from have suggested that I begin my day by asking myself the question, "How can I be of service?" I have found this to be useful in reminding me of the multitude of ways that I can be helpful to others. When I take the time to ask this question, I find answers popping up all day long.

If one of your goals is to be of help to others, you will find the most appropriate ways. Your chances to be of service are endless. Sometimes the best way that I can be of service is to offer my home to someone in need. Other times, it's to give my seat to an elderly person on the train, help a youngster across the monkey bars, speak to a group, write a book, or write a check to a charity. The key, I believe, is to remember that being of service isn't a one-time effort. Instead, a life of service is a lifelong process, a way of thinking about life.

When you give, you also receive. In fact, what you receive is directly proportional to what you give. As you give more freely of yourself in your own unique ways, you will experience more feelings of peace than you ever thought possible.

264.

SHORT-CIRCUIT YOUR REACTION SPIRALS

It's a rare person who can avoid the trap of reaction spirals. This is the insidious tendency to overreact to something—and then compound the problem by overanalyzing it. Here is a typical example: Someone criticizes some aspect of your work. You overreact to the criticism and become defensive. As if that weren't bad enough, you spend the next half hour analyzing the critical comments, convincing yourself they are incorrect.

Wouldn't it be wonderful if you could nip these reaction spirals in the bud? You can! The trick is to see them coming and to commit, in advance, to short-circuiting them. With every negative reaction comes a negative feeling—a feeling of irritation, annoyance, or impatience. We often use these feelings to justify further negativity. If, instead of compounding our negative feelings, we used them as a signal to alert us to potential trouble, we would be in a much better position to stop the cycle before it got out of hand.

Many potential problems can be averted with this simple strategy. All you really need is the wisdom to understand that negative reactions aren't in your best interest, and the humility and willingness to back off and start over. Don't waste your precious energy compounding an already negative situation. You'll be amazed how much smoother your life will become and how easily you can get back on track when you short-circuit your reaction spirals.

265.

DON'T FIGHT OVER STUPID THINGS

This strategy speaks right to the heart of the matter. Fighting over stupid things is another way of saying you're sweating the small stuff—big time! Yet, I see it all the time: couples, families, and friends arguing and bickering over the most ridiculous things. People argue over who misplaced the scissors, whose turn it is to take out the trash, which one of you has more free time, or who works harder! I even know a woman who started a fight because her husband put the towels in the wrong bathroom! What could possibly be more insignificant than that?

When you eliminate (or even greatly reduce) the number of little things that bother you enough to fight about, it opens the door to a different kind of relationship. It's so much fun to be around someone who isn't always bothered by something—it's refreshing, inviting, and nourishing.

Ask yourself the question, "Do I want my life to be about fighting over stupid things and demanding that everyone else, especially the people I love, be different?" By simply asking this question in such a direct and honest manner, the answer will become an obvious . . . no.

266.

STOP PROCRASTINATING

I know plenty of people who are virtually always late, whether it's to pick up the kids in their carpool, sit down before church starts on Sunday, or prepare food for dinner guests. The interesting part of this tendency isn't the fact that they are always running late, but the excuses that are used: "I had to pick up three kids," "I had to make two stops before work," "It's tough to get everything done before I run out the door."

I'm not denying that it is tough to get everything done—it is—but in all of these examples, you are working with absolutely known variables. You know exactly how many kids you have and how long it takes to get them ready. You know how long it takes to drive to work, and that there will be traffic.

To get over this tendency requires humility. The only solution is to admit that, in most instances, you do have the time, but you must start a little earlier. This is one of the simplest suggestions I've made, yet in some ways it's one of the most important. Once you get in the habit of starting a little earlier, a great deal of your daily stress, at least that portion that you have some degree of control over, will fade away.

267.

REMEMBER THE THREE R'S

The three R's that are helpful if you want to learn to be a less reactive, happier person are: Responsive, Receptive, and Reasonable.

"Responsive" means acting appropriately to the issue at hand. Rather than being driven and controlled by habitual, knee-jerk reactions, being responsive means having the ability to maintain perspective and to choose the best possible alternative or course of action, given your unique situation.

"Receptive" implies being open to ideas and suggestions. It means you are willing to receive whatever it is that you need at that moment—data, creativity, a new idea, or whatever. It's the opposite of being closed-minded and stubborn. People who are receptive are willing to have a "beginner's mind," the willingness to learn, even if they are the expert.

"Reasonable" suggests the ability to see things fairly, without the self-serving justification that so often clouds our vision. It's the ability to see your own contribution to a problem and the willingness to listen to and learn from other points of view. Being reasonable includes the ability to put yourself in the shoes of others, being able to see the bigger picture, and to maintain perspective.

If you can strive to be responsive, receptive, and reasonable, my guess is that most everything else will fall into place and take care of itself.

268.

KEEP IN MIND THAT CIRCUMSTANCES DON'T MAKE A PERSON, THEY REVEAL THEM

It's extremely rare to find a successful person who complains and frets about her circumstances. This is despite the fact that she may have overcome great obstacles. On the other hand, it's extremely common for struggling individuals to continually blame their circumstances for their lack of joy. What came first—the attitude or the success? The answer, in virtually all cases, is the positive attitude came first.

Your circumstances are what they are; they were what they were. When you argue for your limitations, your thoughts and words merely get in your way and greatly interfere with your ability to create. With complaining out of the way, you'll create the space for an explosion of creativity and brilliance.

All it takes is a simple decision—the decision to stop yourself from falling into the complaining habit. At first it may be difficult—even funny—to observe how often you complain. Habits can be hard to break. But it's well worth the effort. As an excuse or complaint comes to mind, gently shoo it away like you would flies at a picnic. You'll quickly get used to the nicer feelings that come from a life without complaints, as well as the success that comes with your new winning attitude!

269.

DO A FAVOR AND DON'T ASK FOR, OR EXPECT, ONE IN RETURN

So often, either consciously or unconsciously, we want something from others, especially when we have done something for them—"I cleaned the bathroom; she should clean the kitchen." Or, "I took care of her child last week, so she should offer this week." It's almost as though we keep score of our own good deeds rather than remembering that giving is its own reward.

When you do something nice for someone, just to do it; you'll notice (if you're quiet enough inside yourself) a beautiful feeling of ease and peace. You don't need something in return or even a "thank you." In fact, you don't even need to let the person know what you have done.

What interferes with this peaceful feeling is our expectation of reciprocity. Our own thoughts interfere with our peaceful feelings as they clutter our minds, as we get caught up in what we think we want or need. The solution is to notice your "I want something in return" thoughts and gently dismiss them. In the absence of these thoughts, your positive feelings will return.

270.

GET OUT OF THE GRUMBLE MODE

Grumble, grumble, grumble. Someone who takes himself, others, and everything else too seriously. The primary focus is on problems, always critical, frowning, angry, and defensive. Someone who is waiting for life to get better, for things to be different. Is this you?

While you're in the midst of your career, while there are problems to deal with, it seems as if life is going to last forever. Yet deep down we all know that, in reality, life slips away too quickly. You had your chance to experience and explore life and its many facets—the beauty as well as the hassles. But in a way, you took it for granted. You spent your time grumbling, wishing life were different.

The good news is, it's never too late to change. In fact, once you see how ridiculous it is, you can change quickly.

A grumbler will blame life for his sour attitude. He will validate his negativity by pointing to the problems and hassles that he must face. A grouch can begin to feel better by recognizing the absurdity of a negative attitude. In order to shift from grumble mode to a less serious nature, you'll need to get a sense of humor—the ability to look back at the way you used to be, and chuckle.

271.

STOP WISHING THEY WERE DIFFERENT

There is no question that, philosophically, this is one of the most important strategies in this book. The connection between wishing our partners, children, and friends were different and our own level of dissatisfaction is powerful and significant. To make matters worse, this insidious habit is often invisible to ourselves, or at least is very subtle.

When we love someone, it's tempting and perhaps almost inevitable to fall into the trap of yearning for a slightly "better" version of them. We might wish our loved one were a better provider, more ambitious, a better listener, more passionate, more helpful, or some combination of the above.

The problem is, whenever there is a gap between what we have and what we want, we will feel dissatisfied or frustrated. It's a hard-and-fast rule of life. It's difficult, however, to make this connection because it seems that your lack of satisfaction is coming directly from the person themselves.

As an experiment, take note of your dissatisfactions, the aspects of your loved one that you wish were different. Now ask yourself the questions, "What would happen if I could stop wishing she would change?" "What would happen if I decided to love him just the way he is?" Look for ways to love them as they are. The love you've been waiting to experience is within your own grasp.

272.

THINK OF YOUR PROBLEMS AS POTENTIAL TEACHERS

Problems come in many shapes, sizes, and degrees of seriousness, but all have one thing in common. They present us with something that we wish were different. The more we struggle with our problems and the more we want them to go away, the worse they seem and the more stress they cause us.

Luckily, the opposite is also true. When we accept our problems as an inevitable part of life, when we look at them as potential teachers, it's as if a weight has been lifted off our shoulders.

Think of a problem that you have struggled with for quite some time. If you're like most, you've probably struggled with it, mentally rehearsed it, over-analyzed it, but have come up short. Where has all this struggle led you? Probably to even more confusion and stress.

Now think of the same problem in a new way. Rather than push away the problem and resist it, try to embrace it. Ask yourself what valuable lesson(s) this problem might be able to teach you. Could it be teaching you to be more careful or patient? Does it have anything to do with greed, envy, carelessness, or forgiveness? Whatever problems you are dealing with, chances are they could be thought of in a softer way that includes a genuine desire to learn from them.

273.

GET IT OVER WITH

It's easy to look at your list of things to do and avoid, procrastinate, postpone, or even conveniently forget that which you least want to do.

I've created a habit for myself that has undoubtedly saved me hours of unnecessary stressful or worrisome thinking: I attend to the most difficult or uncomfortable parts of my day first, before anything else, getting them out of the way.

For example, I may have to resolve a conflict, make a difficult phone call, deal with a sensitive issue, engage in a confrontation, turn someone down or disappoint them, or something else that I wish I didn't have to do. I've made a commitment to myself that, whenever possible and practical, I make that phone call first—before anything else. I get it over with!

Without question, saving the most uncomfortable parts of your day for last is an extremely stressful thing to do. The longer you wait, the more likely you are to blow it out of proportion, imagine the worst, and get yourself all worked up.

The simple solution is to dive in and get it over with, whatever "it" happens to be. You'll breathe a sigh of relief when it's over and done with. You can then get on with the rest of your day.

274.

SIMPLE PLEASURES

Kris was talking with a woman about the challenge of sticking to a budget. The woman was telling Kris that she was furious and frustrated that her husband loved to go out to lunch rather than pack a lunch. Her husband's position was quite different. To him, going out to lunch was one of the few things he loved to do for himself. He was stressed at work, and getting away during his lunch hour to a quiet café brought him peace of mind.

I couldn't resist writing about this subject because it's symbolic of something so much greater than the cost of lunch. The question is, "What is a simple pleasure that brings your loved one joy really worth?" To us, the answer has always been, "It's worth a great deal."

There is something magical that happens when you stop insisting on being "right" and instead soften your positions to accommodate those you love. I'm not suggesting that you always have to bend or accommodate your loved one's needs, or that you should do so if the request is truly unreasonable. Yet, when you know something isn't that big a deal, and it makes someone else happy, it might be better for your relationship to allow them to have their way. Give it a try, and your relationships will prosper.

275.

FORM A WINNING PARTNERSHIP

As you probably already know, the wrong partnership—professional or personal—can be far worse than no partnership. And a winning partnership can be worth its weight in gold. Sometimes, however, fear can keep us from seeking out good partners and forming winning partnerships. As always, it's a good idea to overcome this fear so that you will know whether forming a winning partnership is in your best interest.

Ideally, each partner brings to the table different skills and attributes. One might be excellent at details and planning, the other in promotion and public speaking. A good partnership is like a good marriage—it must be formed carefully. If you can create the right combination of skills, work ethic, and vision, you can create a winning team.

What kind of partner do you need to achieve your dreams? This could be support in your life goals (a running partner to train for a marathon), at work (a partner to take your business to the next level), or in your personal development (an accountability partner). You may be the most talented person on earth, but until you hook up with a good partner, you may never truly unleash that talent.

276.

GET COMFORTABLE NOT KNOWING

One day, a farmer from a small village went to the local wise man and said frantically, "Wise man, help me. My ox has died and I have no animal to help me plow my field! Isn't this the worst thing that could have possibly happened?" The wise old man replied, "Maybe so, maybe not."

The next day a strong horse was seen near the man's farm. With no ox to rely on, he caught the horse. He returned to the wise man to apologize. "You were right. Losing my ox was a blessing in disguise! This is the best thing that could have happened." The wise man replied once again, "Maybe so, maybe not."

Later, the farmer's son was thrown from the horse and broke his leg. The farmer returned again. He said, "How did you know my horse was not a good thing? My son is injured and won't be able to help with the crop. This is the worst thing that could have possibly happened." The wise man said compassionately, "Maybe so, maybe not."

The next day troops arrived to conscript every able-bodied man to war. The farmer's son was the only young man in the village who remained.

The moral of this story provides a powerful lesson. The truth is, we don't know what's going to happen—we just think we do.

277.

DON'T PUT PEOPLE ON THE SPOT

Here is a classic example: The phone rings and your partner answers. A mutual friend is calling to ask if the two of you would like to get together over the weekend.

For weeks, you've been looking forward to a quiet weekend and a chance to catch up on some home projects. Your partner, however, is in a social mood and wants to go out.

Here's where it gets sticky. Your partner pulls the phone away from her ear and says to you, "Honey, we're all going to get together this weekend. Doesn't that sound great?" Susan, on the other end of the line, can hear everything you're saying and is now awaiting your response.

Now you're on the spot. You don't have even a single moment to reflect on your priorities or know how to decline graciously. However, there is a solution so simple and respectful that it's a shame not to use it. Philosophically, it might be called, "It's not fair to put my loved ones on the spot." That's it. Problem solved. Everyone wins, no one's feelings are hurt, and no one is put on the spot.

Not always, but usually, you can avoid putting your partner, friends, or family members on the spot. If you do, you'll be rewarded with a more relaxed and probably more loving relationship.

278.

MAKE SOMEONE ELSE FEEL GOOD

One of the first real-life lessons my parents taught me when I was a child is perhaps the most basic of all: if you want to feel good about yourself, make someone else feel good! It really is that simple. Perhaps it is because this idea is so simple that we sometimes forget to do it. It seems that anytime I go out of my way to make someone else feel good, it ends up brightening my day and making myself feel better as well.

Whether it's remembering a birthday with a thoughtful card, taking the time to write a note of congratulations for a job well done, giving a written or verbal compliment, a friendly phone call, an unasked-for favor, a bouquet of flowers, a note of encouragement, or any number of other possibilities, making someone else feel good—however you do it—is almost always a good idea.

There's an old saying: "Giving is its own reward." This is certainly true. Your reward for being kind and making someone else feel good are the warm, positive feelings that invariably accompany your efforts. So, starting today, think of someone you'd like to make feel better and enjoy your reward.

279.

ACKNOWLEDGE THE TOTALITY OF YOUR BEING

Zorba the Greek was said to have described himself as "the whole catastrophe." The truth is, we're all the whole catastrophe, only we wish that we weren't. We deny the parts of ourselves that we deem unacceptable rather than accepting the fact that we're all less than perfect.

Accepting all aspects of yourself allows you to be easier on yourself, more compassionate. When you act or feel insecure, rather than pretending to be "together," you can open to the truth and say to yourself, "I'm feeling frightened and that's okay." When you no longer think of your negative feelings as a big deal, you will no longer be as frightened by them.

When you acknowledge the less-than-perfect parts of yourself, something magical begins to happen. Along with the negative, you'll also begin to notice the positive, the wonderful aspects of yourself that you may not have given yourself credit for, or perhaps even been aware of.

Opening to the totality of your being is like saying to yourself, "I may not be perfect, but I'm okay just the way I am." You may indeed be "the whole catastrophe," but you can relax about it. So are the rest of us.

280.

COMPETE FROM THE HEART

Competition is a fact of life. To pretend that it doesn't exist or that you should avoid it at all costs would be ridiculous. It's been said, "Winning isn't everything, it's the only thing." To me, this is utter nonsense. This philosophy stems from the fear that if you aren't consumed with winning, you never will win.

Instead, competing from the heart means that you compete less from a desperate or neurotic need to achieve and more out of a love for what you do. Competing is its own reward. You are completely immersed in the process, absorbed in the present moments of the activity—the business deal, the sale, the run, or whatever. When you compete from your heart, the process itself provides the satisfaction; winning is secondary.

"Maybe it's just because I'm older now, but I've become much softer," says Mary, a television producer. "Looking back, I realize how incredibly harsh I was, and how unnecessarily mean-spirited I could be. It's weird—but now, I'm just as discriminating and picky as before, but when I have to reject someone, I do so with compassion, without making them feel worse than they already do. I like myself better now, too."

When you compete from the heart in this healthier, more loving way, you get the best of both worlds—achievement and perspective.

281.

LET GO OF FEARFUL THOUGHTS

If you gathered up all the fearful thoughts that exist in the mind of the average person, looked at them objectively, and tried to decide just how much good they provided that person, you would see that all fearful thoughts are useless. They do no good. Zero.

Sometimes fearful thoughts sound reasonable: "I'm just being careful, so I'm taking my time." Other times they are tied to your past: "I've tried that before and it didn't work." Occasionally, fears are cleverly disguised as being realistic: "Most people fail, so I want to be absolutely sure before I begin." All of them are rationalizations for why something shouldn't or can't work. Let me assure you that I'm not suggesting you ignore the facts and take unnecessary or foolish risks. What I'm talking about here are the fears that clearly and directly interfere with your dreams—the fear of rejection, the fear of failure. These common, ongoing fearful thoughts are the dream snatchers of our own making.

Let me suggest you try something that can change your life. Make a commitment that, for the next month, you will practice dropping and ignoring any negative and fearful thought that enters your mind. As they return (which they will), let them go again. It's easier than you think. It just takes courage and a little practice.

282.

BACK OFF WHEN YOU DON'T KNOW WHAT TO DO

It's tempting, when you don't know what to do, to try to force the issue. You try harder, think faster, attempt to figure things out, and struggle to come up with something. You give it your best shot.

The problem is, it usually isn't your "best shot." It seems ironic, yet often the most powerful and productive thing to do when you don't have an immediate answer to a problem is to gently back off of your thinking, consciously ease up, let go, and extend less effort. Doing so frees your mind and allows your innate intelligence and wisdom to come into play.

We mistakenly believe that when we relax, our minds stop working. This is far from true. When we quiet the mind, it's still working—only in a different way. When your mind is active, full speed ahead, it tends to spin and churn. An overactive mind often goes over the same set of facts again and again, encouraging you to think "inside the box."

Somewhere in all the churning of an overactive mind, your wisdom and common sense get lost. These invisible, usually overlooked qualities get buried in a sea of activity, and you fail to see the obvious. I know it seems strange that less effort is better, but it's really true.

283.

CUT YOURSELF SOME SLACK

Each of the strategies in this book is geared toward helping you become more relaxed, peaceful, and loving. One of the most important pieces of this puzzle, however, is to remember that your goal is to stay relaxed, to not get too worked up or concerned about how you are doing. Practice the strategies, keep them in mind, yet don't worry about being perfect. Cut yourself some slack! There will be many times when you lose it, when you revert to being uptight, frustrated, stressed, and reactive—get used to it. When you do, it's okay. Life is a process—just one thing after another. When you lose it, just start again.

One of the most common mistakes I see when people are attempting to become more inwardly peaceful is that they become frustrated by little setbacks. An alternative is to see your mistakes as learning opportunities, ways to navigate your growth and perspective.

All that's important is that, generally speaking, you are doing your best and that you are moving in the right direction. When you can learn to keep your perspective and to stay loving toward yourself, even when you prove you are human, you'll be well on your way to a happier life.

284.

WHEN IN DOUBT, PAUSE

This strategy might appropriately be called an "irritation stopper." Over the years it has helped Kris and me, individually and as a couple, to keep our irritation, annoyance, and frustration with one another to an absolute minimum. It keeps us from turning day-to-day "small stuff" into big stuff.

One of the reasons so many things seem so urgent is that, rather than pausing to reflect, we react instantly to our initial impulse. Our mind latches on to a thought, and we allow ourselves to get carried away.

It's awesome to think about how much time and energy you could save, and how much nicer your relationship could be, if you could eliminate or even reduce these and thousands of other, similar types of reactions. In most instances, all that it takes is a reflective pause. The rest takes care of itself.

It won't always be the case, but most of the time, if you take a moment to pause before reacting, it will allow you to gather your bearings as well as your perspective. Even if something still seems important, it probably won't seem quite so urgent. There's something in the pause itself that creates a sense of peace and allows your wisdom to surface. There's no question that pausing will help you avoid sweating the small stuff.

285.

ADMIT THAT IT'S YOUR CHOICE

The admission I'm referring to is your choice of career and the accompanying hassles. When I suggest that you admit that your job or career is your choice, I'm not saying that your problems are necessarily your fault, or that it's realistic that you make other choices. What I am suggesting is that you have weighed the options, studied the consequences, and you've decided that your best alternative is to do exactly what you are doing.

Megan, a single mother, had a full-time job as a nurse but dreamed of becoming a hospital administrator. When I met her, she confessed to having spent the previous eight years convincing herself that she was a victim. Despite the very real difficulties she was facing, one of her friends had convinced her to stop blaming her circumstances. She listened and had the humility to make the change.

The way she put it: "The moment I admitted that *I* was the choice-maker, everything fell into place. I was able to enroll in the part-time night school program, and I'm already a third of the way through. It's frightening to think about how much I was getting in my own way."

Taking responsibility for your choices takes you out of any "poor me" thinking and into an empowering, "I'm in charge of my own life" mind-set.

286.

LEARN ABOUT MOODS

Moods are one of those unavoidable, mysterious parts of life that must be dealt with by everyone. Our understanding of moods greatly affects not only our wisdom and perspective but our overall level of satisfaction as well. When our mood is high, our spirits are up. When our mood is low, our spirits are down. Moods are like the weather, constantly changing.

The implications of moods as they relate to how we think about our success and security are significant. When we are low, we think of our dissatisfactions more than when we feel good. We worry. We compare ourselves to others and convince ourselves that others are doing better than we are.

When our mood is high, we think very differently. We don't worry as much. Rather than believing that others are doing better than we are, we realize that we are all on different paths, doing the best we can. Instead of seeing people as selfish, we realize that most people are very generous and giving.

So, what do you do? Resist the temptation to worry about your moods. Moods are always changing, and yours could change at any moment. Simply realizing that you are stuck in a mood usually raises your spirits. Again, don't worry! As your mood rises, your capacity to create will unfold.

287.

STOP BLAMING OTHERS

When something doesn't meet our expectations, many of us operate with the assumption, "When in doubt, it must be someone else's fault." You can see this assumption in action almost everywhere you look—something is missing, so someone else must have moved it; the car isn't working right, so the mechanic must have repaired it incorrectly; a project is late, so your colleagues at work must not have done their share—and on and on it goes.

In terms of personal happiness, you cannot be peaceful while at the same time blaming others. Surely, there are times when other people and circumstances contribute to our problems, but it is we who must rise to the occasion and take responsibility for our own happiness. Circumstances don't make a person, they reveal him or her.

As an experiment, notice what happens when you stop blaming others for anything and everything in your life. This doesn't mean you don't hold people accountable for their actions, but that you hold yourself accountable for your own happiness and for your reactions to other people and the circumstances around you. When the house is a mess, clean it up! When you're over budget, figure out where you can spend less money. Most important, when you're unhappy, remind yourself that only you can make yourself happy.

288.

REFLECT, FOR A MOMENT, ON ALL YOU DON'T DO

It's human nature to be focused on what you're doing. It's a way of keeping track of what is being done and what isn't. In a way, it's hard not to do this—your responsibilities are in your face, twenty-four hours a day.

However, if you think about it, there are probably things you don't have to do, at least very often. Whether it's your partner cleaning the house, a friend making a dinner reservation, or a sibling hosting at the holidays, there are many responsibilities that you don't take care of.

The idea isn't to compare who has it easier or tougher, or who is doing more or less. Instead, the idea is to spend a little less time thinking about all that you do—and a little more time reflecting on and appreciating all the things you don't have to do. If you can find even a single thing that you don't have to do—no matter how small it is—you will feel a hint of gratitude. You'll be amazed at how much resentment will fade away, how much less you'll be sweating the small stuff, and how much more you'll appreciate your loved ones by incorporating this exercise into your life.

289.

SURROUND YOURSELF WITH EXPERTS

So many people surround themselves with "successful" people and "experts." Yet they are intimidated by them, frightened that people who are more successful won't be willing to spend time or share their ideas. Nothing could be further from the truth. The reality is, accomplished people love it when someone takes an interest in their success; they love to share their wisdom, good ideas, or business secrets. It makes them feel wanted and needed.

I've worked on projects with some very famous, successful people through some of my other books. When people ask me, "How in the world did you convince them to participate?" they are often shocked at the simplicity of my answer. I respond honestly by saying, "I just asked them."

You'll be amazed at the number of people who are more than willing to help, whether it's the owner of a successful grocery store, a top-producing insurance salesperson, a well-known author, a physician, a lawyer, or an excellent teacher. Most want and are willing to offer advice. In fact, asking someone you admire and respect for their feedback and ideas is the greatest compliment you can offer them.

If you want great advice and you want to avoid big mistakes, seek help. Surround yourself with winners. Go straight to the top.

290.

BEFORE BECOMING DEFENSIVE, TAKE NOTE OF WHAT IS BEING SAID

Essentially, all that this strategy involves is making the decision to step back, breathe, relax, and genuinely listen before you react or feel defensive. That's it. This simple commitment will help keep you from becoming defensive.

Suppose your boss takes a quick look at something you've spent months working on. You've poured your best efforts and many late nights into the project. You're proud of your work and expect that others will be, too. Your boss, however, obviously doesn't appreciate what went into your efforts, nor is she impressed. Her comment is something to the effect of, "Couldn't you have done this differently?"

If you implement this strategy into your reactions, you would in effect create a buffer or space between the comment and your defensive reaction—time for you to gather your composure and perspective. Does the comment make sense? Is there an element of truth in it? Can you learn something here? Or is the person simply being a jerk? The more honestly you can assess the situation, the more helpful it will be.

While it's not always easy, it sure pays huge dividends to take careful note of what is being said—before becoming defensive. If you do, you'll find yourself becoming less defensive on a regular basis.

291.

PRACTICE UNCONDITIONAL LOVE

Unconditional love is perhaps the ultimate expression of love. It says, "I love you because you are you. You don't have to be any different from who you are to receive and secure my love."

Other than our own children (and only then when they are very tiny), it's probable that few of us (if any) will ever love someone entirely unconditionally. Whether we know it or not, we usually place certain conditions on our love (e.g., you must behave in certain ways to secure my love—you must put me first, you must be faithful, you must think like me, prioritize my goals, and so forth).

Despite the fact that we're probably doomed to never reach perfection, we can certainly come much closer to reaching our goal of unconditional love if we set lofty goals. We can "catch ourselves" when we become judgmental or behave in unkind ways. We can strive to become less jealous and demanding and replace those tendencies with gratitude and softness. Or we can become better listeners and be more forgiving.

You can be sure that whatever efforts you make to become a more unconditionally loving person, you will see results in the quality of your relationships. This is one of those strategies where you have absolutely nothing to lose—and everything to gain.

292.

BECOME AN EARLY RISER

So many people wake up, rush to get ready, grab a cup of coffee, and charge out the door to work. After working all day, they return home, tired. The same is usually true for those who stay home with their children. Whether you work, raise a family, or both, for the most part you are too tired to enjoy any time left for you. As a solution to the tiredness, the assumption is often made, "I'd better get as much sleep as I can." So, your free time is spent sleeping. For many people this creates a deep longing in the heart. Surely, there must be more to life than work, children, and sleep!

Another way of looking at your fatigue is to consider that a lack of fulfillment and a sense of being overwhelmed both contribute to your tiredness. And contrary to popular belief, a little less sleep and a little more time for you might be just what you need to combat your sense of fatigue.

An hour or two that is reserved just for you—before your day begins—is an incredible way to improve your life.

Many people have told me that this one shift in their routine was the single most important change they have ever made in their lives.

293.

FULLY COMPLETE AS MANY TASKS AS POSSIBLE

Most people don't understand how stressful it can be to have multiple incomplete tasks hanging over your head. I like to call this the "almost finished syndrome." It has always intrigued me because often it would be relatively easy to simply hunker down and complete something—not almost complete something, but really complete it 100 percent, and get it out of the way.

When you absolutely finish a project, several good things happen. First, you enjoy the nice feeling of a sense of completion. It feels good knowing you've set out to do something and it's done, it's out of the way. Completion allows you to move forward without the distraction of having things hanging over your head.

Beyond the obvious, however, is the respect you feel for yourself and the respect you secure from others when you complete something. You said you were going to do something, and you did it—all of it. You send the message to others that "I am a person of my word." And you affirm the message to yourself.

Take an honest look at your own tendencies. If you are someone who often *almost* finishes something, take note of the tendency and commit yourself to that last, final step to completion. You can do it—and when you do, your life is going to seem so much easier.

294.

DON'T MAKE ANYONE WALK ON EGGSHELLS

There are many consistent comments that people make regarding what frustrates them in their relationships. Near the top of this list is the complaint, "I feel like I have to walk around on eggshells."

What a shame! You're in a relationship that is supposed to be mutually satisfying, and you're constantly worried that your loved one is never more than seconds away from losing it, or from expressing some kind of disappointment, directed at you.

As you read these paragraphs, ask yourself the question, "Are there ways that I encourage others to feel they must walk around on eggshells?" If you find yourself answering "Yes," it may be time to reevaluate your priorities and perhaps even lower your expectations a little bit.

If you're not sure whether you're contributing to this problem, just ask. Really!

This is one of those hard-to-admit but easy-to-fix habits that occur in many relationships. The first step is to see that it's in everyone's best interest if no one has to feel like they must walk around on eggshells. After that, the solution becomes paying attention to your own feelings of frustration. When you begin feeling tense, remind yourself to lighten up. Put things in perspective.

295.

WHEN TRYING TO BE HELPFUL, FOCUS ON LITTLE THINGS

Mother Teresa once said, "We cannot do great things on this earth. We can only do little things with great love." Sometimes our grandiose plans to do great things interfere with our chances to do little things right now. A friend once told me, "I want my life to be about service, but I can't do anything yet. Someday, when I'm really successful, I'll do lots of things for others." Meanwhile, there are hungry people in the streets, elderly people who could use some company, parents who need help with their children, streets with litter, people who need to be listened to, and thousands of other little things that need to be done.

We can't change the world, but to make the world a brighter place, we don't need to. All we really have to do is focus on those little acts of kindness, things we can do right now. Often, the most appreciated acts of kindness aren't the million-dollar grants from giant corporations but the one hour of volunteer work in a home for the elderly or the five-dollar gift from someone who can't afford anything at all.

If we take great care in doing something—anything—we will feel the joy of giving and will help to make our world just a little bit brighter.

296.

SPEND TEN MINUTES A DAY DOING ABSOLUTELY NOTHING

I'll bet you're already thinking, "I could never do that," or "What a waste of time." If so, I'm happy to tell you that you're off base on both counts. I absolutely understand how busy you must be, and I'm certain beyond any doubt that ten minutes of doing absolutely nothing can be the most productive ten minutes of your entire day.

For most of us, a typical workday is sort of like a horse race—the moment we're out of bed, the race has begun. Collectively, we're so busy that when the slightest glitch occurs or when something goes wrong, we fall apart and feel frustrated.

When you sit still and do nothing, it allows your mind the opportunity to sort things out and settle down. It turns what usually looks like chaos into a more manageable moment and provides your mind with a chance to rest and regroup. When you're finished doing nothing or sitting still, it will often seem like life is coming at you a little slower, which makes everything seem a whole lot easier and less stressful.

At first glance, this concept may seem counterproductive. Yet one of the most powerful and sure ways to achieve even more success in your life is to do absolutely nothing for a few minutes a day.

297.

THE CRITICAL INCH

Often, the greatest mistake people make in their quest for success is focusing on the wrong work. Part of the solution is asking the relevant question: "What's truly most important?" Often, the answer is quite different from the answer to another question: "What seems to be the next logical or convenient thing to do?"

You can see the same principle at the gym. There are some people who show up, roll up their sleeves, and get to work. Then there are people who chat for a bit, take twenty minutes to get changed, and walk around the gym looking at the equipment. Recently, I overheard a phone conversation between a man and his partner. He said, "Honey, I just don't get it. I go to the gym virtually every day, without results." Now, I've seen this man at the gym on many occasions, but I've yet to see him actually work out. He never seems to do the critical inch—the exercise!

If we're not careful, it's easy to fall into the same basic trap in many spheres of our lives. We may look busy and do quite a few things during the course of a day, but we might not be focusing on the one or two things that really make a difference.

298.

USE LETTERS AS A COMMUNICATION TOOL

Typically, when you confront someone, or when you need to have a serious discussion, it can be difficult to fully articulate your position and why it matters to you without the other person becoming at least slightly defensive. Before you have fully laid out your argument, they are already sharing (or at least thinking about) their concerns and comebacks.

Therefore, in certain situations, writing a letter can be a powerful way to overcome this problem. A nondefensive and "from the heart" letter can be a wonderful way to communicate a concern, preference, or potential solution.

As the writer, you have the chance to think about and describe your position slowly and carefully, without the chance of being interrupted. The recipient of the letter has the advantage of being able to read the letter as many times as is needed in order to fully understand where you are coming from.

Such letters are not intended to be a substitute for honest and courageous communication. They are best used to open the door to relationship-deepening communication. As long as the letter is written with love, respect, and sincerity, it's hard to imagine that it wouldn't be well received.

299.

REMEMBER, ONE HUNDRED YEARS FROM NOW, ALL NEW PEOPLE

My good friend Patti recently shared this bit of wisdom with me that she learned from one of her favorite authors. It has added a great deal of perspective to my life.

In the scheme of things, one hundred years isn't all that long a time. However, one thing's for sure: a hundred years from now we will all be gone from this planet. And when kept in mind, this idea can fill us with needed perspective during times of perceived crisis or stress.

If you have a flat tire or lock yourself out of your house, what's it going to mean one hundred years from now? How about if someone acted unkindly toward you or if you had to stay up most of the night working? What if your house didn't get cleaned or your computer breaks down? All of these things and most others are brought into a deeper perspective when looked at with a hundred-year view.

Just this morning I found myself at a mental fork in the road, about to get uptight about a mini crisis at work. What saved me from getting overly stressed and too uptight was remembering that one hundred years from now, no one will remember this moment, no one will care.

300.

LEAVE A GREAT IMPRESSION (NOT JUST A GOOD ONE)

When people have a nice feeling toward you, it sets you apart. This doesn't mean you should pretend to be someone you're not, only that you recognize that your presence, behavior, integrity, and kindness will leave a lasting imprint in the minds of those you are with.

The way to do this is very simple. Make living your life with absolute integrity and kindness your priority. Put others first, whenever possible. Be genuinely interested in the lives of other people. Be very present-moment oriented with others. Look them in the eye and really focus on what they're saying. Care about them as individuals. Ask about their families. Listen, listen, listen. Finally, make your actions match your good intentions. Stand out from the crowd. Be the one to thank those around you and the people with whom you work. Make people remember you in a positive light.

If you implement this strategy with your own unique touches and if you are genuine in your thoughts and actions, you will create a stellar reputation with virtually everyone you meet. What's more, your life will be filled with more joy and loving-kindness than you ever thought possible.

301.

LEARN TO DELEGATE

I've found that many people—even very high-achieving, talented, and successful people—are often very poor delegators. The feeling is, "I might as well do it myself—I can do it better than anyone else." There are several major problems with this attitude. First of all, no one can do all things or be two places at once.

Often, it not only helps you but someone else when you delegate at work. When you ask for help, share responsibility, or delegate authority, you are often giving someone a chance to show you, or someone else, what they can do. I know that a cynic will say, "The only reason people delegate is to shove off the tough and dirty work on others." And, yes, there are plenty of people who look at it that way—but you don't have to. The point is, there are good reasons—in addition to selfish ones—to practice delegation.

Whether at work or at home, chances are there are some places where you can let go and delegate a task. If you think about your specific circumstances, you'll probably be able to think of at least a few ways to become a better delegator. If you do, you'll free up some time and make your life easier.

302.

PRACTICE REGULAR STRESS PREVENTION

Many of the most effective things you can do to become happier and more peaceful fall into a category that we like to call "stress prevention."

Stress prevention involves any activity or attitude that is designed (or tends) to produce, on its own, a calmer and more accepting attitude toward life.

I once did an informal research study project to determine the effectiveness of various stress-reducing techniques. What I discovered was impressive but not surprising. People who took a regular yoga or meditation class (once a week) were three times less likely to describe their relationships as being "stressful." And even when they did complain about their relationships, the complaints were usually minor and discussed with a sense of humor and perspective. There was a slightly less dramatic, yet similar statistic for people who exercised regularly and took care of themselves, who took time out to relax or to read, or who spent time praying, congregating with like-minded people, or reflecting.

Taking some time each day, whenever possible, to attend to your inner self, and to cultivate a sense of well-being, however you do it, pays enormous dividends in your personal life and in your relationships. Explore, investigate, and try out your many stress-prevention options. When you're happy and relaxed, life tends to appear pretty darn good.

303.

LIGHTEN UP

These days, it seems that almost all of us are too serious. My older daughter often says to me, "Daddy, you've got that serious look again." Even those of us who are committed to nonseriousness are probably too serious.

The root of being uptight is our unwillingness to accept life as being different, in any way, from our expectations. We want things to be a certain way, but they're not a certain way. Perhaps Benjamin Franklin said it best: "Our limited perspective, our hopes and fears become our measure of life, and when circumstances don't fit our ideas, they become our difficulties."

The first step in recovering from overseriousness is to admit that you have a problem. You have to want to change, to become more easygoing. You have to see that your own uptightness is largely of your own creation.

The next step is to understand the link between your expectations and your frustration level. Whenever you expect something to be a certain way and it isn't, you're upset and you suffer.

A good exercise is to try to approach a single day without expectations. Don't expect your day to be problem free. Instead, as problems come up, say to yourself, "Ah, another hurdle to overcome." If you approach your day in this manner, you'll notice how graceful life can be.

304.

ELIMINATE YOUR MOST SELF-DEFEATING BELIEF

All of us have beliefs that get in our way. And for many of us, there is one in particular—some nagging, habitual tenet that we have come to accept. For me, it was my belief that "I don't have enough time." Day after day, I would remind myself of this limiting concept.

There is no value in this kind of limiting belief. Consider the subtle messages that go along with this idea. After all, if I believe that "I don't have enough time," I must also believe that "I'll never get anything done on time," "I'll be under constant pressure," as well as other related ideas that directly interfere with my quality of life.

What's *your* most self-defeating belief? Is it that you believe you aren't good enough or lucky enough? Maybe you believe you don't deserve success, or that other people control your destiny. Whatever it is, it's not worth keeping, and it's certainly not worth defending!

Each time I slip into my old habit of telling myself that I don't have enough time, I keep in mind the damage I am inflicting on myself. You'll be pleasantly surprised at how easily you can rid yourself of the negative effects of a defeating idea. Simply refuse to continue. Without these limiting beliefs, you'll discover that joy is right around the corner.

305.

STRENGTHEN YOUR PRESENCE

Presence is a magical quality that is difficult to define. In fact, it's easier to describe its absence. In other words, you can usually tell in an instant the difference between someone who has it and someone who doesn't. A person with powerful presence is said to be charismatic and magnanimous—people are drawn to his or her energy.

Having a strong presence does not necessarily mean you are outgoing, although it might. It's more a matter of being centered in yourself, comfortable with who you are, and completely absorbed in the moment. When you have a strong presence, the people you are with sense that you are truly "right there" with them, fully present. Your mind isn't drifting somewhere else.

When you have presence with others, they are drawn to you. They relax around you and become less defensive. They enjoy your company and feel your sincerity; they feel important when they are with you.

The way to strengthen your presence is to understand its value. Make an ongoing effort to stop your mind from wandering. When you are with someone, be with them. When your mind wanders, gently bring it back. Try to have more presence, see it as a worthwhile goal, and it will appear in your life.

306.

REMEMBER THE HAPPINESS EQUATION

Sometimes, the most obvious equations are the most overlooked. This strategy falls into this category. For whatever reasons, we often choose personal convenience or some other selfish reaction over attempting to look after the happiness of our partner or other loved ones. Yet doing so violates a clear equation—a happy person equals a happy relationship—and pretty much guarantees unnecessary stress and strife.

I'm certainly of the mind-set that it's not your responsibility to make others happy. In fact, there's an entire strategy in this book dedicated to the idea that we all must take responsibility for our own happiness. Yet there are things all of us can do—little things, no-brainers—that clearly contribute to our loved one's happiness. A happy person is also more likely to be a better listener and a more passionate lover, more inclined to share in the joy of others, more giving and compassionate, and more likely to make decisions that enhance the quality of a relationship.

So, what's the catch? The catch is that, occasionally, it's inconvenient to make decisions that make your partner happy. Or it requires a little sacrifice. Or it makes you a little uncomfortable. But in the end, it's almost always worth it.

307.

NURTURE A PLANT

At first glance this may seem like a strange suggestion. What good could it do to nurture a plant?

One of the goals of spiritual life and one of the requirements of inner peace is to learn to love unconditionally. The problem is, it's really hard to love a person, any person, unconditionally.

A plant, however, is easy to love just the way it is. Therefore, nurturing a plant offers us an excellent opportunity to practice unconditional love.

Select a plant, indoor or outdoor, that you will see every day. Practice taking care of and loving that plant as if it were your baby (it's easier to care for your plant than your baby—no sleepless nights, no diapers, no crying). Talk to your plant. Love your plant whether it blooms or not, whether it lives or dies. Just love it. Notice how you feel as you offer this plant your unconditional love. When you offer this type of love you're never agitated, irritated, or hurried. You're simply in a loving space. Practice this type of love each time you see your plant, at least once a day.

Soon, you'll be able to extend your loving-kindness beyond your plant as well. As you notice how good it feels to love, see if you can offer a similar love to the people in your life.

308.

STAY COMPASSIONATE

To be compassionate means you strive to know what it's like to be in the shoes of another person. Generally, we feel compassion when we see someone suffering; we want to reach out to them—to be a source of support, help, love, or understanding. Compassion is one of the beautiful characteristics that make us human. The more compassion we feel and express, the more human we become.

There is something strange, however, that seems to occur in most relationships—especially long-term ones. Gradually, over time, we lose our compassion for our partner, friend, or family member. Somehow, we begin to see them in a different light than we do others—we take them for granted and forget, or lose sight of, the fact that they are human, too, and are subject to the same pain and suffering as everyone else.

Stay compassionate, and your relationships will be on solid, loving ground. If you have lost your compassion, however, or if it's slipping away, you can get it back. All it takes is a simple reminder that your loved one's pain is every bit as real as anyone else's. He or she is subject to the same fears, feelings, doubts, and concerns as everyone else. Daily compassion strengthens your love and mutual respect for one another like nothing else.

309.

LEARN TO SAY NO WITHOUT GUILT

One of the ways that many of us get ourselves into trouble is that we commit to too many things; we fail to say no.

The problem with always saying yes is twofold. First, the result is almost always feeling overwhelmed, stressed, and tired. By saying yes too often, we begin to feel victimized and resentful that we have so much to do.

The second major problem with failing to say no is that you end up with a slightly disingenuous attitude. In other words, you are doing things you really don't want to be doing or shouldn't be doing—but you are acting, on the surface, as if everything is just fine.

Saying no without guilt is not selfish—it's a protective necessity. If someone said to you, "Can I have the air you breathe?" you'd probably question their sanity. You certainly wouldn't feel guilty saying no.

Obviously, there are many times that we can't say no, and many other times when yes is the right answer. Terrific! The key is to be reflective and to ask yourself, "All things considered (e.g., the feelings and needs of the person making the request, the need to say yes, and most important, my own sanity), is it in my best interest to say yes, or is it okay to refuse?"

310.

TRANSFORM YOUR RELATIONSHIP TO YOUR PROBLEMS

Obstacles and problems are a part of life. True happiness comes not when we get rid of all of our problems, but when we change our relationship to them, when we see our problems as a potential source of awakening, opportunities to practice patience, and to learn. Perhaps the most basic principle of spiritual life is that our problems are the best places to practice keeping our hearts open.

In the Buddhist tradition, difficulties are considered to be so important to a life of growth and peace that a Tibetan prayer actually asks for them. It says, "Grant that I may be given appropriate difficulties and sufferings on this journey so that my heart may be truly awakened and my practice of liberation and universal compassion may be truly fulfilled." It is believed that when life is too easy, there are fewer opportunities for genuine growth.

I wouldn't go so far as to recommend that you seek out problems. I would, however, suggest that you spend less time running away from problems—and more time accepting problems as an inevitable, natural, even important part of life. This philosophy of acceptance is the root of going with the flow.

311.

TAKE YOUR NEXT VACATION AT HOME

Here's a scenario. You finally get a week off. You have a great trip planned, yet you still have to do all that's necessary to leave. You rush to pack and to get all the loose ends sorted out. You're exhausted. Yet here you are, running to catch another airplane.

Part of you can't wait for your adventure—but the other part would love the chance to piddle around the house, curl up with a great book, start that yoga or exercise program, or maybe take a couple of simple, but relaxing day trips closer to home.

Kris and I had a great home-based vacation several years ago. Work was off-limits, we hired a babysitter in the mornings, ordered takeout, and spent the time doing yoga, finishing home projects, playing as a family, being in the garden, and just unwinding. The kids had a blast, and so did we.

I'm not advocating replacing all traditional vacations. I love to go away, and I suspect you do, too. I can tell you, however, that this is a great way to relax, as well as a chance to do things you almost never get to do at or close to home, while spending very little money.

312.

CHOOSE TO BE SUPPORTIVE (KRIS)

Every relationship will have its share of ups and downs. However, you can keep the inevitable downs from spiraling ever further downward by choosing to be supportive.

Trish and Gavin had been married for ten years when, quite unexpectedly, Gavin lost his job. With two young children and a hefty mortgage, there was genuine cause for alarm.

The way Trish handled this crisis was courageous and filled with wisdom. Scary as it was (and it really was), she made the decision to remain supportive. Rather than complain or belittle Gavin in even the slightest way, she made it perfectly clear that she would do whatever was necessary to support him in his efforts.

While many people may also have responded to such a crisis by being supportive, what made her response so unique was her uplifting attitude. She wasn't being supportive with a hint of resentment. Rather, her support was genuine and from the heart.

We can all learn from their experience and the way Trish handled herself. We don't always have control over our destiny—but we do have some control over the way we choose to respond to adversity.

313.

DON'T LIVE IN AN IMAGINED FUTURE

If you want to be a happier, less-stressed person, there is no better place to start than with becoming aware of what I like to call "anticipatory thinking," or an imagined future.

Typical anticipatory thinking goes something like this: "I can't wait to get that promotion, then I'll feel important." "My life will be so much better when my 401k is fully funded."

Or more short-term forms of this type of thinking, like: "The next few days are going to be unbearable," or "I just know my meeting is going to be a disaster." You get so carried away by your own thoughts that you remove yourself from the actual present moments of your life, thereby postponing the act of living effectively and joyfully.

Whether you're dreading tomorrow's meeting, or next year's obstacles, the trick is to observe your own thoughts caught up in the negative expectations and imagined horrors of the future. Once you make the connection between your own thoughts and your stressful feelings, you'll be able to step back and recognize that if you can rein in your thoughts, bringing them back to what you are actually doing—right now—you'll have far more control over your stress level.

314.

THE NEXT TIME YOU FIND YOURSELF IN AN ARGUMENT, RATHER THAN DEFEND YOUR POSITION, SEE IF YOU CAN SEE THE OTHER POINT OF VIEW FIRST

When you disagree with someone, the person you are disagreeing with is every bit as certain of his or her position as you are of yours. Yet we always take sides—ours! This is our ego's way of refusing to learn anything new. It's also a habit that creates a lot of unnecessary stress.

The first time I consciously tried this strategy, I found out something truly wonderful: it didn't hurt, and it brought me closer to the person with whom I was disagreeing.

Suppose a friend says to you, "Liberals [or conservatives] are the major cause of our social problems." Rather than automatically defending your own position (whatever it is), see if you can learn something new. Say to your friend, "Tell me why you think that's true." Don't say this with a hidden agenda or in preparation to defend or prove your position. Don't try to correct or make your friend see how he is wrong. Practice being a good listener.

Contrary to popular belief, this attitude does not make you weak. It doesn't mean you aren't passionate about your beliefs, or that you're admitting that you're wrong. You're simply trying to see another point of view—you're seeking first to understand.

315.

DON'T LET NEGATIVE PEOPLE GET YOU DOWN

Learning to deal with negative people is a real art form, but I can tell you with absolute certainty that it's well worth the effort. Consider your options. If you don't do what's necessary to deal gracefully with negative people, you may end up cynical and negative.

The best place to start is by increasing your level of compassion. It's critical to see the innocence, to understand that when someone is negative, they are unfulfilled or in some way unhappy. They would prefer to experience contentment and joy. They just don't know how.

One of the reasons negativity tends to bring us down is that we take it personally or we feel that we are in some way responsible. When viewed with compassion, however, it's easy to see that negativity is usually not directed at us, even if it appears to be.

Your best chance of distancing yourself from the effects of negativity is to remain enthusiastic yourself, therefore being part of the solution rather than contributing to the problem. Instead of focusing on how hard it is to be around a negative person, try instead to be genuinely enthusiastic about your work and about your life in general. In all likelihood, you will have a significant effect on the negative people you work with.

316.

DON'T FORGET TO HAVE FUN

When you look back on your life, perhaps on your deathbed or toward the end, it's very likely that you *won't* be asking yourself how much money you made or how many possessions you managed to collect. Nor will you see the purpose of life as being the collection of achievements or even the fulfillment of your goals. What you will see, I believe, is that the purpose of life was to have been kind and loving, to grow and to give back to others. You will have plenty of regrets if you forget to have fun, and probably none if you do not.

Realizing your dreams—whatever they are—can be a blast. It's certainly enjoyable to feel financially secure or successful, but even more so to use your mind, attitude, charm, wisdom, and genuine kindness to create great abundance in all aspects of your life.

The more fun you have, the more you are likely to succeed. This is your life. You have the right to enjoy it. So be successful and create great abundance, but don't forget to have fun!

317.

REDEFINE A "MEANINGFUL ACCOMPLISHMENT"

If you ask the average person (as I have done many times), "What is a meaningful accomplishment?" the typical responses will be things like "achieving a long-term goal," "earning lots of money," "getting a promotion," "being the best," "earning praise," and so forth. The emphasis is almost always on the external aspects of life—things that happen outside of ourselves. Certainly, there is nothing wrong with these types of accomplishments—they are ways of keeping score and improving our circumstances. They are not, however, the most important types of accomplishments if your primary goal is one of happiness and inner peace.

If being peaceful and loving are among your primary goals, then why not redefine your most meaningful accomplishments as being those that support and measure qualities such as kindness and happiness?

I think of my most meaningful accomplishments as stemming from inside myself: Was I kind to myself and others? Did I overreact to a challenge, or was I calm and collected? Am I happy? Did I hold on to anger or was I able to let go and move on? Was I too stubborn? Did I forgive? These questions, and others like them, remind us that the true measure of our success comes not from what we do, but from who we are and how much love we have in our hearts.

318.

MAKE THE BEST OF A "NONCREATIVE" POSITION

I wanted to include this strategy because I've spoken to so many people over the years who complain about their "noncreative" position or yearn for a more interesting job.

You have a choice regarding any job that you might consider to be noncreative. You can dread each day and wish it were different. Or you can remind yourself, "It is what it is," and go ahead and make the best of it. You can be enthusiastic and have a positive attitude. You can find ways to make the job as interesting as it can possibly be. You'll be at work for the same number of hours either way.

I've met toll-takers who have told me that their job isn't to take money from people, but to see how many people they can make smile.

I've found that those people who approach their job in this positive way are almost always the ones who enjoy their work the most—and usually the ones who move quickly up the ladder if that is what they choose to do. Their attitude is lighthearted and relaxing to themselves, and inspiring and contagious to others.

If you've gotten in the habit of thinking only certain jobs and careers can be fun, give it some more thought. When you make the best of it, almost anything can be "creative."

319.

DON'T CONFUSE YOUR FRUSTRATION WITH A PROBLEM IN YOUR RELATIONSHIP

It's human nature, when you're frustrated, to try to figure out why you're feeling so bad and pinpoint blame. So, when you're sad, you may think, "If I only knew why I was so upset, I'd start to feel better." Then it hits you! "That's it—I know what it is—my relationship has some problems!" Immediately, you get into detective mode and think of all the ways your relationship isn't what it should be.

If you step back from this tendency, however, you'll begin to see that it's precisely because you are frustrated that problems and issues in your relationship are coming to mind. Out of the frustration came the tendency to see, create, and analyze problems. This isn't to say that the problems you notice when you're feeling bad are not real. However, if a problem is legitimate, it will certainly still seem that way when you're feeling good.

Not always, but most of the time the problems that look so real and significant when you're feeling low magically disappear when you're in a better frame of mind. It happens much of the time. When you're feeling down, don't take your thoughts and feelings as seriously. When you're feeling down, you have less wisdom, compassion, perspective, and common sense.

320.

MAKE PEACE WITH CHAOS

One of my favorite "to the point" quotes is from Wallace Stegner. It reads, "Chaos is the law of nature. Order is the dream of man."

Indeed, chaos is the law of nature. It's everywhere you look. People are coming and going, trends come and go, there are unlimited conflicting interests and desires, and change is constant and inevitable.

Despite this undeniable law of nature, we would love to be able to keep things the same, predict our future, keep a perfect balance, and know the answers. But no one can make perfect sense of chaos because it doesn't really make sense—it just exists.

By easing up on your need to control your environment or predict certain outcomes, you're able to learn to work within an environment of chaos without being as affected by it. You begin to experience chaos with a degree of equanimity, with a sense of humor and perspective.

The trick seems to lie in the willingness to embrace the chaos. In other words, surrendering to the way things really are instead of insisting that things be a certain way.

I've found that there are enough challenges in life to contend with, without also fighting and struggling against things that can't be controlled or avoided. Chaos is on top of this list.

321.

WORK AT IT

Perhaps the most difficult insight about building a life of success in work is that, although it's fun and simple, you do have to work on it. These dreams, although within the grasp of anyone, do not necessarily come naturally.

We can break tasks into two basic categories. There are those tasks we know we have to study and learn, and then there are those that just come naturally. To build a suspension bridge obviously requires a lot of specific learning, and breathing comes naturally at birth. Now, here's the question: "Does abundance come naturally, like eating and breathing, or is it a task that must be learned and worked at?" I think it's a little of both.

It's a natural process, but it does take some work. The best and most empowering ideas are simple, but they require implementation. I believe I am empowering you when I tell you that it's your choice. Once you have insight about your part in the process, you can open the door and do something about it. This is a powerful and important door to open. You have the power to create the life of your dreams. Go ahead and make it happen!

322.

LISTEN TO YOUR FEELINGS (THEY ARE TRYING TO TELL YOU SOMETHING)

You have at your disposal a foolproof guidance system to navigate you through life. This system, which consists solely of your own feelings, lets you know whether you are off track and headed toward unhappiness and conflict—or on track, headed toward peace of mind. Your feelings act as a barometer, letting you know what your internal weather is like.

When you're not caught up in your thinking, taking things too seriously, your feelings will be generally positive. They will be affirming that you are using your thinking to your advantage.

When you're feeling angry, resentful, depressed, stressed out, frustrated, and so forth, your warning system of feelings kicks in like a red flag to remind you that you are off track.

The next time you're feeling bad, rather than getting stuck in "analysis paralysis," see if instead you can use your feelings to guide you back in the direction toward serenity. Don't pretend that the negative feelings don't exist, but try to recognize that the reason you're feeling sad, angry, stressed, or whatever is that you are taking life too seriously—you are "sweating the small stuff." Instead of rolling up your sleeves and fighting life, back off, take a few deep breaths, and relax. Remember, life isn't an emergency unless you make it so.

323.

STAY CLOSE TO YOUR CENTER

You can think of your center as home base, your most natural way of being. When you're centered, you have the sense that you're flowing, on target, and in the groove. You have the feeling that you're on track, that you'll be able to work things out, solve your problems, and get your work done.

On the other hand, when you're off-center, you are filled with frightened, scattered, agitated, and other stressful feelings. You feel pressured and off-balance, as if there's not enough time.

Staying close to your center isn't as difficult as you might imagine. It involves paying attention to your feelings and gently bringing yourself back when you start to drift away. For example, you might be working on a project when your attention drifts forward in anticipation of your deadline or you begin to imagine negative responses to your work.

You're at an important fork in the road. If you continue with your train of thought, it's likely that you will continue to feel agitated, pressured, and even resentful. If you observe what's happening, you can choose to back off your thinking for the moment in order to get back closer to your center.

Staying close to your center is in your best interest. I encourage you to explore this idea, work with it, and enjoy the rewards.

324.

DON'T FALL INTO THE "I'VE GOT TIME FOR EVERYONE BUT YOU" TRAP

I've seen this easy-to-fall-into trap hurt so many relationships that it's almost painful to write about. As most of us know all too well, it's easy to get overwhelmed with all the responsibilities of life, to fall short of time and find ourselves scrambling, in desperate need of cutting back our schedule.

Unfortunately, without even knowing it, it's often our loved ones who get pushed to the back of the line. In other words, in our efforts to get everything done, we end up neglecting the people we love most in the world—our partner, children, or others we love deeply. Sadly, when we do, we put a hurtful wedge between ourselves and those we love.

Obviously, we do have tremendously busy lives. But it's important to become aware of this tendency—and to see how easily it can happen. Even though you may love someone more than anything in the world, the messages you are sending may contradict this love. The adage "Actions speak louder than words" is really true.

There may be no perfect way to completely overcome this tendency—I sure haven't found one. However, it's enormously helpful (on a regular basis) to honestly reflect on your relationship and see where this habit may already be sneaking in.

325.

ASK YOURSELF, "WHAT HAVE I CONTRIBUTED TO THIS PROBLEM?"

Many people rarely, if ever, ask this critical question. Instead, they automatically assume that any problem they are having must be someone else's fault. If there is a disagreement or argument, it's the other person's fault. If there's a glitch in the schedule, someone else must have dropped the ball. It simply never occurs to many people that something is *their* fault.

The problem with this "never blame me" philosophy is that you'll rarely be able to pinpoint the one aspect of problem-solving that is truly solvable: your own contribution. Once you eliminate the fear associated with admitting that you are, at times, responsible for the parts of your life that aren't working—minor annoyances and larger problems—you open a whole new door of possibilities.

Once you're willing to accept responsibility for the problems in your life, you will see obvious solutions that take very minor adjustments to change. Sometimes there's a fine line between doing something really well and doing something really badly.

Obviously, I'm not suggesting that everything is your fault, or that you should spend an exorbitant amount of time and energy thinking about your faults and drawbacks. It's critical, however, that you're at least honest about your contribution to your problems.

326.

WHEN SOMEONE THROWS YOU THE BALL, YOU DON'T HAVE TO CATCH IT

My best friend, Benjamin Shield, taught me this valuable lesson. Often, our inner struggles come from our tendency to jump on board someone else's problem; someone throws you a concern, and you assume you must catch it and respond. For example, suppose you're really busy when a friend calls in a frantic tone and says, "My mother is driving me crazy. What should I do?" Rather than saying, "I'm really sorry, but I don't know what to suggest," you automatically catch the ball and try to solve the problem.

Remembering that you don't have to catch the ball is a very effective way to reduce the stress in your life. When your friend calls, you can drop the ball, meaning you don't have to participate simply because he or she is attempting to lure you in. If you don't take the bait, the person will probably call someone else to see if they will become involved.

This doesn't mean you never catch the ball, only that it's your choice to do so. Neither does this mean that you don't care about your friend, or that you're crass or unhelpful. Developing a more tranquil outlook on life requires that we know our own limits and that we take responsibility for our part in the process.

327.

FORGIVE YOURSELF; YOU'RE HUMAN

I've never understood why a simple fact of life—our tendency to make mistakes—is so surprising or disappointing to people. I certainly don't understand why it's such a big deal.

To me, one of the saddest mistakes we make is a lack of forgiveness, especially to ourselves. We constantly remind ourselves of our flaws and previous mistakes. We anticipate future mistakes. We're highly critical of ourselves, frequently disappointed, and ruthless in our self-judgment.

I'm sure that one of the reasons I'm a happy person is that I'm very forgiving of my mistakes. Someone recently asked me how I learned to be so kind to myself. My response was, "Because I've made so many mistakes, I've had lots of practice."

Obviously, some mistakes are big. An air traffic control mistake or one wrong move by a surgeon can be deadly. Most of the mistakes we make, however, are not life or death; they are nothing more than "small stuff" disguised as "big stuff."

While no one enjoys making mistakes, there is something very freeing about learning to accept them—really accept them—as an unavoidable part of life. When we do, we can forgive ourselves, thus erasing all the stress that usually results from badgering ourselves. So my suggestion is simple: forgive yourself. You're human.

328.

ONE MORE PASSING SHOW

This strategy is a subtle reminder that everything—good and bad, pleasure and pain, approval and disapproval, achievements and mistakes, fame and shame—comes and goes. Everything has a beginning and an ending and that's the way it's supposed to be.

Every experience you have ever had is over. Every thought you've ever had, started and finished. Every emotion and mood you've experienced has been replaced by another. You've been happy, sad, jealous, depressed, angry, in love, shamed, proud, and every other conceivable human feeling. Where did they all go? No one really knows. All we know is that, eventually, everything disappears into nothingness. Welcoming this truth into your life is the beginning of a liberating adventure.

Our disappointment comes about in essentially two ways. When we're experiencing pleasure we want it to last forever. It never does. Or, when we're experiencing pain, we want it to go away—now. It usually doesn't. Unhappiness is the result of struggling against the natural flow of experience.

It's enormously helpful to experiment with the awareness that life is just one thing after another. One present moment followed by another present moment. Keeping this awareness close to your heart is a wonderful way to maintain your perspective, even in the face of adversity. It's not always easy, but it is usually helpful.

329.

BE PROCESS ORIENTED

Many of us have a tendency to be "list oriented." Someone who is list oriented feels good when something is taken off his list—and feels annoyed or frustrated when there is an obstacle that prevents him from doing so.

If you're list oriented, for example, and you're working on a project, you're going to feel good only when the project or sale is complete—and only if it meets your expectations. But what if things don't work out according to plan? And even if they do, what about all the time between the start of the project and the result? The work itself, including the hassles, obstacles, and disappointments, is what life and work are all about. Therein lies the bulk of your time.

A different approach is to view your day-to-day experiences, tasks, and responsibilities not only as items to be checked off your list but rather as part of a process; to see it all as necessary and interesting. Rather than focusing on and being driven only by the result, you become interested in the entire experience—however it happens to unfold.

So, whatever it is that you do for a living, see if you can become less attached and zeroed in on the result or outcome and, instead, become more engaged in each moment along the way.

330.

TURN UP THE HEAT

In theory, if your home was too cold, there would be two ways to warm it up. The first would be to walk around the house making sure the windows were tightly closed; you'd check the weatherstripping, the insulation in the attic, and any cracks in the walls, gaps around the edges of doors, and so forth. In doing so, you'd keep additional outside cold air from entering the house. The other, more direct (and much quicker) approach would be to simply turn up the heat. Bingo—in a matter of a few minutes, your home would be warm and cozy—regardless of any tiny cracks.

You can easily extend this metaphor to your relationships with others. You can attempt to create warmth and closeness by fixing everything that's wrong. But like heating a home, a more direct (and more effective) approach would be to (metaphorically) turn up the heat—you become kinder and more generous, and you start dishing out more compliments. You become less critical, stubborn, and judgmental. Instead of being irritated, you practice patience and forgiveness.

If you turn up the heat in this way, your relationships will blossom even though there are tiny flaws. In fact, with enough warmth, most flaws and imperfections will work themselves out without much involvement or effort.

331.

MARVEL AT HOW OFTEN THINGS GO RIGHT

Have you ever, even once, stopped to marvel at just how often things go right? It's amazing. Literally thousands of events—work related and otherwise—go right every single day, without a glitch. Everything from the vast majority of phone calls that are returned and reservations that are honored, to travel and food safety, dependency on various forms of technology, roofs that don't leak, the competency of coworkers, the interdependence of schedules, right down to the fact that most people are friendly—so much goes right. And for the most part, we take it all for granted.

I'm not going to discount the fact that there are problems to deal with; there most certainly are. It seems that we've become so accustomed to things going smoothly, however, that we expect near perfection. When we don't get it, we go crazy.

I think it's wise to keep at least a little bit of perspective. When I remind myself of how often things actually go right, it really helps me deal with those things that don't. It allows me to make allowances for the fact that "stuff happens," people make errors, Mother Nature does her thing, and things do sometimes go wrong.

332.

FILL YOUR LIFE WITH OPPORTUNITIES TO EXPRESS LOVE

It has been said that "the shortest distance between two points is an intention." This is certainly true with regard to a life filled with love. The starting point or foundation of a life filled with love is the desire and commitment to be a source of love. Our attitude, choices, acts of kindness, and willingness to be the first to reach out will take us toward this goal.

The next time you find yourself frustrated at the lack of love in your own life or at the lack of love in the world, try an experiment. Forget about the world and other people for a few minutes. Instead, look into your own heart. Can you become a source of greater love? Can you think loving thoughts for yourself and others? Can you extend outward toward the rest of the world—even to people whom you feel don't deserve it?

By opening your heart to the possibility of greater love, and by making yourself a source of love (rather than getting love) as a top priority, you will be taking an important step in getting the love you desire. Soon you'll discover one of the greatest secrets in the world: love is its own reward.

333.

LET GO OF YOUR TOP THREE PET PEEVES

For years, I've been asking the question, "What is it that bugs you the most about your partner?" There are two broad themes that stand out. First, more often than not, what bugs people are the little things. Second, on average, there seem to be about three primary pet peeves per person.

There are only two ways to overcome this reality. The first is pure fantasy—thinking that the other person is going to be able and willing to change. But the other way is incredibly effective—to let go of your top three pet peeves.

This sounds harder than it actually is. When you examine your options, you'll discover that this is indeed your best course of action. You'll see that the reason pet peeves bug you is that you allow them to bug you.

One of my previous pet peeves with Kris was that she frequently forgot to turn off her closet light. It's a stupid little thing that used to drive me nuts! Then one day it hit me. If this was all I had to complain about Kris—I'm one really lucky guy! I hope you'll agree that choosing to let go of your top three pet peeves is a good idea. Who knows, perhaps your loved one will let go of something irritating about you!

334.

THE IDEA THAT "OPPORTUNITY ONLY KNOCKS ONCE" IS A MYTH

It's hard to imagine a belief that is based more on fear than this one. Yet this idea is so common to our collective consciousness that it has turned into a cliché. When people believe this idea, it's as if they're saying to themselves and to the world, "My creative days are over. I'm a complete package. My life has been lived out." Nonsense!

Opportunity exists virtually everywhere you look. There are books that need to be written, children who need to be taught, houses that need to be built, people who need help. So many people can benefit from and need our unique creativity. We live in a world of unlimited potential, a world of creative genius.

If you buy into the belief that opportunity only knocks once, you may jump on board too quickly when something that looks like an opportunity presents itself. You may take a job that you don't really like, or move to a location that doesn't suit your temperament. Instead of picking and choosing wisely, from a place of wisdom, joy, and common sense, you may end up reacting impulsively.

Let go of your fear. The universe has an infinite supply of opportunity. You may be surprised to see that something is coming your way right now.

335.

PREVENT BURNOUT

There's no way to guarantee the prevention of burnout, but there are things you can do to put the odds in your favor.

The keys seem to be balance and growth. If you talk to people who aren't burned out, you'll discover that most of them strive to have a balanced life and to be growth-oriented.

When all you do is work, burnout will be the result. Think about it. What would happen if you only ate one food, year after year? It wouldn't matter if it was your favorite food or not—you'd get sick of it.

This is a strategy that some people try to dismiss with the old excuse, "I don't have time to have a life." Unfortunately, this is a narrow and extremely short-sighted way of looking at your life and your career. The truth is, for most people, if you don't "get a life," you will end up with a major case of burnout.

Start by evaluating your priorities apart from work. If you had to pick, what would be most important? Would it be to volunteer? Is it your spiritual life? Would it be to schedule a regular date with your partner, your child, or a friend? Or something else entirely? Whatever it is, take a look at your calendar and begin to carve out the time. Anything is better than nothing.

336.

ORGANIZE A CHARITABLE PROJECT

In the flurry of everyday life, it's easy to get caught up in our own worlds—to become frustrated by the demands of life. And while there's no question that life can be frustrating, even overwhelming at times, it's equally true that doing something for others or for a cause we believe in helps to reduce that frustration. By putting some of our attention on "doing good," and a little of our effort and time into something other than our own "stuff," we remind ourselves that there's more to life than meets the eye—that our problems, especially the small ones, can usually be put into perspective. We get to experience the pure joy of giving—of seeing something through, start to finish, that is purely positive and unselfish, something that has nothing to do with "us," or with our ordinary day-to-day existence.

Kris and my first project together was a grassroots food drive. Despite the fact that our project was extremely small by almost any standard, and completely unsophisticated in nature, planning it turned out to be a significant moment in our lives. It was then that we dedicated our lives to kindness and service. We saw how incredibly easy it was to do something for others and how much joy it brought to our lives and to our relationship.

337.

REALIZE THE POWER OF YOUR OWN THOUGHTS

If you were to become aware of only one mental dynamic, the most important one to know about would be the relationship between your thinking and the way you feel.

Try getting angry without first having angry thoughts! Okay, now try feeling stressed out without first having stressful thoughts—or sad without sad thoughts—or jealous without thoughts of jealousy. You can't do it—it's impossible. The truth is, in order to experience a feeling, you must first have a thought that produces that feeling.

Unhappiness doesn't and can't exist on its own. Unhappiness is the feeling that accompanies negative thinking about your life. In the absence of that thinking, the unhappiness, or stress, or jealousy can't exist. There is nothing to hold your negative feelings in place other than your own thinking. The next time you're feeling upset, notice your thinking—it will be negative. Remind yourself that it's your thinking that is negative, not your life. This simple awareness will be the first step in putting you back on the path toward happiness. It takes practice, but you can get to the point where you treat your negative thoughts in much the same way you would treat flies at a picnic: you shoo them away and get on with your day.

338.

EXPERIENCE A MAGICAL TRANSFORMATION

A magical transformation is like a new beginning. It involves extricating yourself from an old, worn-out way of thinking or behaving, and replacing it with a more positive alternative. The transformation itself occurs out of the blue, often when you least expect it.

It might involve giving up a destructive habit or addiction, or it might be a matter of recognizing a self-defeating pattern of behavior or attitude and somehow seeing how to change it.

The easiest way to experience a transformation is to mentally review your most negative traits and habits, the ones you know you'd like to change, and to make a mental note that you'd like to see it differently. I was once sitting with a man who, in the midst of our conversation, had the sudden realization that he was virtually always critical. It was as if he saw it for the first time. I remember him saying, "I can't believe I've always been that way."

Experiencing a magical transformation involves recognizing that you do, indeed, have a choice. Once you are aware that magical transformations are possible, you begin to look for them in your own life.

339.

DON'T SWEAT OCCASIONAL CRITICISM

Sometimes, when someone is criticized, you'd think by their reaction that we were in the midst of a national crisis!

We're all going to get our fair share of criticism during our lifetime. And, if we're in a relationship, at least some of that criticism is going to come from our partner. So, it's unrealistic—in fact, probably a little unfair—to expect that your loved ones won't, at times, criticize you.

When someone criticizes you, it doesn't mean they don't love you. Nor does it mean they don't respect or admire you. Sometimes we criticize out of habit; other times it's because we're frustrated, confused, stressed out, or insecure. Occasionally, we even criticize because we see a flaw that really does need to be fixed. Criticism can be constructive, even helpful.

The best way to deal with occasional criticism is to make allowances for it, and accept the fact that it is going to be directed at you from time to time. It's like rain. You know it's going to come; you just don't know exactly when and under what circumstances. And just like you wouldn't get mad at rain, you don't need to be concerned about small amounts of criticism. All you need to do is allow it to be there—accept it, and let it go.

340.

GIVE UP ON THE IDEA "MORE IS BETTER"

We live in the most affluent culture the world has ever seen. It seems to me that if more were actually better, we would live in the happiest, most satisfied culture of all time. But we don't. Not even close. In fact, we live in one of the most dissatisfied cultures on record.

It's not that having a lot of things is bad, wrong, or harmful in and of itself, only that the desire to have more and more and more is insatiable. As long as you think more is better, you'll never be satisfied.

It's gotten to the point that when the Dalai Lama won the Nobel Prize for Peace, one of the first questions he received from a reporter was "What's next?" It seems that whatever we do—buy a home or a car, eat a meal, find a partner, purchase some clothes, even win a prestigious honor—it's never enough.

The trick in overcoming this insidious tendency is to convince yourself that more isn't better and that the problem doesn't lie in what you don't have, but in the longing for more. Learning to be satisfied doesn't mean you can't, don't, or shouldn't ever want more than you have, only that your happiness isn't contingent on it.

341.

ASK, BUT DON'T INSIST

There's an old saying: "If you don't ask for what you want, you're not going to get it." And while this isn't always the case, from a certain perspective it does make a great deal of sense.

The only problem with the "be willing to ask" philosophy is that it doesn't take into consideration the many times that you don't get something, even when you do ask or when you feel you deserve it. So, the old saying, if taken literally, can create some frustration.

Any potential frustration, however, can be prevented by including a lack of insistence upon your desired result. In other words, it's terrific, courageous, and important to ask for what you want, but if you're attached to the outcome, you could be in for a long and ongoing series of disappointments in your life. Once you detach from the outcome, however, you'll win either way. You'll either get what you want or you'll be okay with the fact that you didn't.

The key to becoming less attached to the outcomes of your requests is to depersonalize them. In other words, try to see that more often than not, being turned down has very little to do with you.

Be sure to ask for what you want, but don't insist on getting it.

342.

REMEMBER THE WHOLE STORY

As you probably know, it's extremely seductive to focus primarily on the negative. But is this negative assessment the whole story—or is it only part of it? Are you recharacterizing your day the way it actually was—or are you being selective in what you choose to remember and discuss?

I encourage you to be completely honest with yourself as you ponder the following questions about your day: On your way to work, did you stop for a bagel and coffee? Did you take a lunch break? If so, who were you with? How was the food? Did you have any stimulating conversations during the day? Any new insights? Did you have a chance to express your creativity? Did you see any pretty sights or nature—trees and flowers, birds or animals? Did you hear any good jokes today? Did anyone give you a compliment? Did you listen to any good music in the car? Did you resolve any conflicts? Are you being paid?

Since I began focusing more on the best parts of my day, my eyes have been opened to a whole new world. I've become increasingly aware that there are all sorts of interesting and enjoyable aspects to my day that were virtually invisible to me prior to this shift in focus. I'm sure the same will be true for you.

343.

KEEP ASKING YOURSELF, "WHAT'S REALLY IMPORTANT?"

As part of my early morning routine, I take a few seconds to ask myself, "What's really important?" Reminding myself of what's really important helps me keep my priorities straight. It reminds me that, despite my multitude of responsibilities, I have a choice of what is most important in my life and where I put my greatest amount of energy—being available for my wife and children, writing, practicing my inner work, and so forth.

Despite the appearance of being overly simplistic, I have found this strategy to be immensely helpful in keeping me on track. When I take a few moments to remind myself of what's really important, I find that I'm more present-moment oriented, in less of a hurry, and that being right loses its appeal. Conversely, when I forget to remind myself of what's really important, I find that I can quickly lose sight of my priorities and, once again get lost in my own busyness.

If you regularly take a minute to check in with yourself, to ask yourself, "What's really important?" you may find that some of the choices you are making are in conflict with your own stated goals. This strategy can help you align your actions with your goals and encourage you to make more conscious, loving decisions.

344.

DON'T OVERANALYZE THE FLAWS

If you overanalyze the flaws of your loved ones, you will be successful in identifying them. You'll be able to convince yourself that they have some serious work to do! In other words, if you look carefully enough, you will succeed in validating the fact that the person you love is riddled with flaws. The more you analyze, the more likely it will be that you'll fall into the "analysis paralysis" trap—the tendency to overuse your thinking.

The problem with this almost insidious tendency is that it virtually guarantees that your relationships will suffer. Most of us are bright individuals. When we look for something—i.e., think about it enough—we will almost always find what we're looking for.

You'll notice, if you reflect carefully, that whenever you overanalyze anything that bothers you, you'll end up a little discouraged or angry. At an absolute minimum, you'll be sweating the small stuff! I think you'll agree that these are not feelings that are ideally suited to bring forth greater love in your relationships.

The next time you find yourself overanalyzing your relationship, see if you can back off. Ask yourself the question, "Am I really upset about my partner/friend/child—or is the fact that I'm totally caught up in my thinking contributing to my unloving feelings?" You may be amazed at what you discover!

345.

NEVER WRITE AN E-MAIL WHEN YOU'RE MAD

I'm borrowing this idea from my wife, Kris, who has written about it in her book, *Don't Sweat the Small Stuff for Women*. It's so pertinent and important to maintaining strong business relationships, avoiding unnecessary conflict, and having a great life that I couldn't resist writing about it here.

It's tempting, when you're mad or upset, to fire off a message that you might very well live to regret. In a reactive or upset state of mind, or when you're lacking judgment or perspective, it's easy to act impulsively rather than with composure and wisdom. In the blink of an eye, you can confuse someone, hurt their feelings, enrage them, or even destroy a relationship.

The good news is that the flip side of this issue is also true. If you're mad at someone and are tempted to share your feelings via e-mail—but you manage to resist—your restraint can pay enormous dividends.

Some practical advice is this: whenever possible, when you're upset, refrain from sending e-mails. It's dangerous territory. Instead, wait until you cool off. Most of the time, what ends up being said will be more rational and will be better received by the recipient.

346.

TAP INTO YOUR SECRET STRESS-BUSTER

Years ago I was home one night scrambling to finish a work-related project that was due the next day. I was uptight, stressed, hurried, and agitated.

A wise friend was visiting from out of town. He looked at me very compassionately and said, "Richard, are you breathing?" Shocked and a little annoyed by what I believed to be a superficial question, I replied, "Of course I'm breathing, aren't you?"

He put his hand on my chest and showed me what I was doing. It was one of the most surprising moments of my life. I was breathing so superficially, it was almost as if I weren't breathing at all!

To my great surprise, as I began to take slightly deeper breaths, I felt instantly better. My body seemed to relax and my thinking became clearer.

Have you ever seen a professional basketball player right before they shoot an important, pressure-packed free-throw? In most instances, the athlete takes a long, deep breath before taking the shot. What I'm suggesting in this strategy is that you incorporate deeper breathing into your everyday work life.

Check in with your breath. How deep is your inhalation? Notice what happens when you consciously breathe just a little deeper. If you're like me, you'll instantly feel more relaxed and less stressed.

347.

TRUST YOUR INTUITIVE HEART

How often have you said to yourself, after the fact, "I knew I should have done that"?

Trusting your intuitive heart means listening to and trusting that quiet inner voice that knows what it is you need to do, what actions need to be taken, or changes need to be made in your life. Many of us don't listen to our intuitive heart for fear that we couldn't possibly know something without thinking it through, or for fear that legitimate answers could possibly be so obvious.

If you can overcome your fear that your intuitive heart will give you incorrect answers, if you can learn to trust it, your life will become the magical adventure it was meant to be. Trusting your intuitive heart is like removing the barriers to enjoyment and wisdom.

If you're unfamiliar with trusting your intuition, start by setting aside a little quiet time to clear your mind and listen. Ignore and dismiss any habitual, self-defeating thoughts that enter your mind and pay attention only to the calm thoughts that begin to surface. If you find that unusual yet loving thoughts are appearing in your mind, take note of them and take action. Start trusting your intuitive heart today and you'll see a world of difference in your life.

348.

GO AHEAD AND DO IT

With the dozens of daily responsibilities that most of us are expected or required to do, it's inevitable that at least a few things are going to slip through the cracks—you'll leave some laundry on the floor or forget to pick up dinner like you promised.

One of the ways we create problems and ill feelings in our relationships is by silently demanding that our loved ones never slip up. We say things like, "You forgot to do the dishes" as if the other person is a robot needing reprogramming. In reality, the person you love is simply a person, who innocently forgot, or was too tired or too preoccupied to take care of it.

Usually, a more effective and less abrasive way to relate to these slip-ups is to simply go ahead and do it yourself—not with any resentment—but rather quietly, selflessly, and lovingly. In other words, if the dishes in the sink are bothering you, wash them.

I'm not asking you to roll over and allow yourself to be taken advantage of. Rather, it's a matter of recognizing that life is complicated, chaotic, and demanding. Very few people feel they have enough time, and almost everyone feels that they have too much to do. Try extending grace to the people you love, and you'll find greater harmony in your relationships.

349.

ENCOURAGE CREATIVITY IN OTHERS AND HAVE FAITH IN THEM

You'd be amazed at what people can (and will) do if you not only give them a chance but also believe in their potential. It's important to know that everyone has unique gifts and talents. It's your job to assist in bringing those gifts and talents out into the world. In other words, rather than sitting back and waiting for people to be perfect—and being frustrated when they are not—take some responsibility in the process by creating an ideal psychological environment.

There's an old motto in business: "Give someone a reputation to live up to and watch them shine." It's true. Most people, given the right environment, are hardworking, talented, creative, and productive.

When you encourage creativity in others and have faith in them, it's analogous to creating the ideal conditions for a garden. You are "planting the seeds" for an environment where success is most likely to occur. When you plant a garden, you want to have the right type of soil, moisture, and sunshine. When you build people up—instead of pushing them down—you create the psychological equivalent.

It always works. When you believe in someone and when that person knows that you believe in them, magical things can happen.

350.

SPEAK TO OTHERS WITH LOVE AND RESPECT

A wise man once told me a story of an unexpectedly pivotal interaction he had at a car wash. The man felt the work on his car hadn't been performed correctly and ended up taking out his frustration on the manager, yelling and chewing him out. The manager agreed to fix the issue and then, in a compassionate but firm voice, he said, "I have to ask you, sir. What makes you think you have the right to speak to me or anyone in that harsh, demanding manner?"

He was stunned and embarrassed, realizing that nothing gave him that right. The man told me that he has spent the last twenty years trying to live up to what he learned that day—remembering that everyone deserves to be treated with respect, no matter what.

When I observe others who are rude, demanding, or insensitive to a flight attendant, a stranger, waitress, grocery clerk, or whomever, I often ask myself the question: "What gives this person the right to speak like this?"

It's always seemed to me that if someone is doing his job, and I'm one of the beneficiaries of their performance, that's all the more reason to speak to him with gratitude and respect. If you're looking for ways to make your life less stressful, this is one of the keys.

351.

ALLOW OTHERS THE SPACE TO "LOSE IT" EVERY ONCE IN A WHILE

It doesn't matter who you are, there are probably going to be times when life just plain gets to you. There is something so refreshing and freeing about being with someone who allows you the space to "lose it" every once in a while—without judging you, correcting you, or trying to talk you out of it. When you're in the presence of someone who doesn't freak out when you freak out, there is often a calming transference that takes place.

The next time your loved one "loses it," try this experiment. Rather than becoming upset or overly concerned about your partner's frustration, just stay calm. Be compassionate, yet don't react. Allow them to vent, yell, complain, or anything else (within reason) that they seem to need to do.

In many instances, they may sense your peace of mind and begin to relax. Often, when people express their frustration, there is a sense that it's not okay to do so. If you can remain relatively unaffected, they may feel a sense of relief that they were listened to without judgment and were given the space to be human. It's strange because you don't have to do anything—except be there for them. In fact, it's more a matter of what you don't do that's ultimately so powerful.

352.

BE OPEN TO "WHAT IS"

One of the most basic spiritual principles in many philosophies is the idea of opening your heart to "what is" instead of insisting that life be a certain way. This idea is so important because much of our internal struggle stems from our desire to control life, to insist that it be different than it actually is.

When we have preconceived ideas about the way life should be, they interfere with our opportunity to enjoy or learn from the present moment. Rather than reacting to a child's complaining or your spouse's disapproval, try opening your heart and accepting the moment for what it is. Make it okay that they aren't acting exactly the way you would like them to. Take a deep breath and soften your response.

You open your heart in these ways, not to pretend that you enjoy complaints, disapproval, or failure, but to transcend them—to make it all right with you that life isn't performing the way you planned. If you can learn to open your heart in the midst of the difficulties of daily life, you will soon find that many of the things that have always bothered you will cease to be concerns. Your perspective will deepen. This is a truly powerful way to live.

353.

DON'T GO THERE

"Don't go there" is an expression that essentially means you know that if you continue on a certain path—thinking in a certain way, arguing, inquiring, discussing, behaving, or whatever—it's going to lead to a predictable, negative result, guaranteed. So, very simply, don't do it! Stop. Don't continue.

For example, you might be asking someone personal questions and notice that he is getting increasingly defensive and angry. If there is no actual reason you need the answers to your questions, this might qualify for the "don't go there" wisdom. The same idea applies to so many interpersonal issues. Often, we know deep down what's going to happen. Sometimes it's best to just "not go there."

I once had a friend who was about to have an affair. He asked me what I thought. My exact words to him were, "Don't go there." For whatever reason, he didn't, and he and his wife were able to improve their marriage.

The simplicity of this expression carries a great deal of power. There are many instances where as simplistic as it may seem, "not going there" is really solid advice.

354.

EMBRACE THE OBSTACLES

The essence of sweating the small stuff is treating life itself as if it were an emergency. Of course, there are emergencies to deal with in life—and they are always difficult. But for the most part, the ordinary, day-to-day, moment-to-moment events, challenges, interactions, and responsibilities we must attend to don't fall into this serious category.

No one is calm all the time, or even close to it. However, it's important to put things into perspective and realize that many of the things we get upset and bothered by aren't really that big a deal but rather just part of our daily lives.

One of my favorite quotes speaks so well to this issue. It comes from Alfred D'Souza. He said, "For a long time it seemed to me that life was about to begin—real life. But there was always some obstacle in the way, something to be gotten through first, some unfinished business, time still to be served, a debt to be paid. Then life would begin. At last it dawned on me that these obstacles were my life."

When we see the obstacles, even the hassles we experience, as an integral part of our life—instead of something that is getting in the way of our life—it makes virtually everything much easier to deal with.

355.

DON'T GIVE AWAY YOUR POWER

A major mistake made by many is to give away one's power to perceived experts. We do it all the time—to our doctors, financial planners, insurance salesmen. The assumption is: This person is an expert, so I'd better listen to her. And, of course, sometimes this assumption is true, and you should listen. But be careful to reserve the ultimate decision-making for yourself.

As usual, the reason we so readily give our power away to others is fear. We worry that if we don't listen to an "expert," then we will surely be making a big mistake. When you make decisions from a place of wisdom rather than from a place of fear—and when you hold on to your own power—your decisions are usually good ones. They take you in directions that lead you toward your dreams and goals. It's a good idea to surround yourself with experts and to understand where your knowledge and experience are limited. However, the power should remain with you.

The ultimate decision is yours. Trust in your own instincts and wisdom, and not in the words and fears of experts. If you have a strong sense that your own instincts are the way to go, follow them. Trust yourself.

356.

MIND YOUR OWN BUSINESS

How often do you find yourself saying things like, "I wouldn't do that if I were her," or "I can't believe he did that," or "What is she thinking about?" How often are you frustrated, bothered, annoyed, or concerned about things that you not only cannot control or be of actual help with but are also none of your business?

This is not a prescription to avoid being of help to people. Rather, it's about knowing when to help and when to leave something alone. I used to be the type of person who would jump in and try to solve a problem without being asked. Not only did my efforts prove fruitless, they were also almost always unappreciated, and sometimes even resented.

Minding your own business goes far beyond simply avoiding the temptation to try to solve other people's problems. It also includes eavesdropping, gossiping, talking behind other people's backs, and analyzing or trying to figure out other people. One of the major reasons most of us focus on the shortcomings or problems of others is to avoid looking at ourselves.

When you catch yourself involved where you really don't belong, congratulate yourself for having the humility and wisdom to back off.

357.

BECOME AWARE OF THE THOUGHT FACTOR

My good friend Joe Bailey was involved in an interesting experiment. He interviewed dozens of drivers during rush hour traffic. Traffic is often included on stress tests designed to quantify how stressed out you must be. At best, traffic is tolerated; at worst, it's cause for road rage. Joe's goal, however, was to show people that, in fact, our thinking, not the traffic itself, is ultimately responsible for the feelings that are experienced in traffic.

The responses to being stuck in horrible traffic were as varied as the types of cars being driven. As you might expect, a certain percentage of drivers were incensed. Others were accepting and relaxed. Some of them used the time to listen to audiobooks or talk on the phone. And believe it or not, a few actually reported that being in traffic was their favorite time of the day—it was the only time they had to be completely alone, slow down, and relax.

This experiment shows us that our experience of life does, in fact, come from our own thinking and perception. If you carefully consider this, you'll see some powerful implications. It means that you really do have a choice in how you respond—not only in traffic, but also in all those other situations that are almost always associated with misery and stress.

358.

LOOK FOR THE EXTRAORDINARY IN LIFE

The truth is, we see in life what we want to see. If you search for ugliness, you'll find plenty of it. If you want to find fault with other people, your career, or the world in general, you'll certainly be able to do so.

But the opposite is also true. If you look for the extraordinary in the ordinary, you can train yourself to see it. The question is: Can you? Can you see the extraordinary synchronicity that exists in our world; the perfection of the universe in action; the extraordinary beauty of nature; the incredible miracle of human life?

To me, it's all a matter of intention. There is so much to be grateful for, so much to be in awe about. Life is precious and extraordinary. Put your attention on this fact and little, ordinary things will take on a whole new meaning.

359.

EASE OFF YOUR EGO

I think of the ego as that part of us that needs to stand out and be special. And while each one of us is certainly special and unique, our ego has the need to prove this to everyone. The ego is that part of us that brags, exaggerates, criticizes, and judges others (as well as ourselves). Because the ego is so self-preoccupied and selfish, it encourages us to lose our compassion for and interest in others.

In addition, the ego is an enormous source of stress. Think about how much energy it takes to prove yourself, show off, and defend your actions. Consider how stressful it is to compare yourself to others. Think about how draining it is to constantly be keeping score of how you're doing and to be concerned with what others think about you.

The first step to easing off your ego is to have the desire to shrink your ego down to size and to see how destructive it can be. The rest is easy. All it takes is humility and patience. When you notice yourself in your "proving mode," gently remind yourself to back off. Be sure to laugh at and be easy on yourself. Don't make letting go of your ego become yet another contest with yourself. It's not an emergency. Be patient and it will happen.

360.

ALLOW YOUR LOVED ONES TO BE HUMAN

At the heart of Kris's and my friendship, love relationship, and marriage is our acceptance of and conscious embracing of the fact that we are two human beings doing the very best that we can. It's true that we love and respect each other—very much—and we are committed in every sense of the word, till death do us part. Yet we both understand that we're just two ordinary people.

Sounds remarkably obvious, and it is. Yet how many people forget this oh-so-important fact of life? How many of us become angry, jealous, or resentful when our loved ones turn out to be none other than human? How many of us are more tolerant and patient with complete strangers than we are with people close to us?

There is something remarkably freeing and magical about seeing loved ones as human beings instead of demanding something that isn't realistic or, we believe, even desirable. It brings back your friendship, shared humanity, and interest in one another.

A question we often ask ourselves and each other is this: "What's wrong with being human, anyway?" Presumably, that's why we're here—to experience being human, to grow, to become more spiritual, to love, and to learn.

361.

CULTIVATE HUMOR AND LEARN TO SMILE

Are you as amazed as I am at all the sourpusses out there in the "real world"? A lot of people have lost their perspective and take life so dreadfully seriously. Everything is a really big deal. On the other hand, once in a while you run into someone who is simply a delight. A person who has cultivated a sense of humor and hasn't forgotten how to smile.

This is undoubtedly one of the simplest suggestions in this entire book. Yet very few understand just how important it really is.

There is a small, family-owned grocery store in our town that is a beneficiary of this philosophy. The owner is one of the nicest men I've ever met. My kids actually ask if we can go to his store, and often we do. There is nothing in his store that we can't get elsewhere—and probably less expensively—but we really prefer to visit him. He has a beautiful smile, and both my daughters and I deeply appreciate it.

Having a sense of humor gives you the privilege of feeling better yourself and making others happy as well. I believe that smiling gives you more energy, and perhaps even better health. So, lighten up and smile. Your payback will be immediate and significant.

362.

SCHEDULE TIME FOR YOUR INNER WORK

In the field of financial planning, there is a universally accepted principle that it's critical to pay yourself first, before you pay your other bills. The rationale for this financial wisdom is that if you wait to put money into savings until after everybody else is paid, there will be nothing left for you!

The identical principle is critical to implement into your program of spiritual practice. If you wait until all your chores, responsibilities, and everything else is done before you get started, it will never happen. Guaranteed.

I have found that scheduling a little time each day as if it were an actual appointment is the only way to ensure that you will take some time for yourself. How you choose to use the time is up to you. The important thing is that you do schedule the time and that you stick to it.

I had a client who actually hired a babysitter on a regular basis to ensure that she had the chance to do the things she felt she needed to do. Today, more than a year later, her efforts have paid enormous dividends. She's happier than she ever thought possible. If you set your mind to it, you can find the time you need.

363.

REMEMBER, SMALL STUFF HAPPENS

Small stuff happens. Even to this day, when I get frustrated over the barrage of small stuff that I have to deal with, my dad reminds me of a quote that, perhaps, says it all: "Life is just one thing after another." How true! You get through one hassle, and another one is just around the corner. You resolve a conflict and inadvertently begin another. You solve a problem and, like magic, another one presents itself. One person is delighted at your performance and in pleasing him, you irritate someone else. Your plans fall through, an error is committed, your computer crashes. It's all part of life, and it's not going to change.

There's something incredibly peaceful in recognizing and surrendering to the fact that small stuff does happen, and that the nature of life is that it's full of conflicting choices, demands, desires, and expectations. Once you stop demanding that life be different, however, the nature of the game changes and you regain control over your life. The same things that used to drive you crazy no longer do. What used to cause you grief, you now see with perspective. Rather than wasting your valuable energy banging your head against walls, you remain calm, deal with the issue as best you can, and move forward.

364.

SAY THE WORDS "I'M SORRY"

I asked an acquaintance of mine a very direct question. It was, "How often does your partner say the words, 'I'm sorry'?" Her answer explains the necessity of this strategy. Her answer was, "You're kidding, right?"

Since then, I have talked to hundreds of people from all over the country. Much to my surprise, not all but most of the people I've asked also reported that the words "I'm sorry" were a minimal, if not practically nonexistent, part of their relationships.

Saying you're sorry, when appropriate, is an extremely healing and nurturing thing to do. It's seen by the recipient not as a sign of weakness, but of strength. It clears the air and opens the door to forgiveness and a fresh start. It brings trust, integrity, and humility into a relationship, three of the most beautiful qualities people can share.

Whether it's over major things or everyday minor things, saying the words "I'm sorry" will usually work to your advantage. It's one of those ever-so-important phrases to introduce to your relationships.

365.

LIVE THIS DAY AS IF IT WERE YOUR LAST! IT MIGHT BE!

When are you going to die? In fifty years, twenty, ten, five, today? Last time I checked, no one had told me.

The truth is, none of us has any idea how long we have to live. Sadly, however, we act as if we're going to live forever. We postpone the things that, deep down, we know we want to do—telling the people we love how much we care, spending time alone, visiting a good friend, taking that beautiful hike, running a marathon, writing a heartfelt letter, going fishing with your daughter, learning to meditate, becoming a better listener, and on and on.

I felt it appropriate to end this book by suggesting that you live each day as if it were your last on this earth. This is not a prescription to be reckless or to abandon your responsibilities, but to remind you of how precious life really is. A friend of mine once said, "Life is too important to take too seriously." Ten years later, I know he was right. I hope that this book has been, and will continue to be, helpful to you. Please don't forget the most basic strategy of all: Don't sweat the small stuff! I will end this book by sincerely saying, "I wish you well."

ABOUT THE AUTHORS

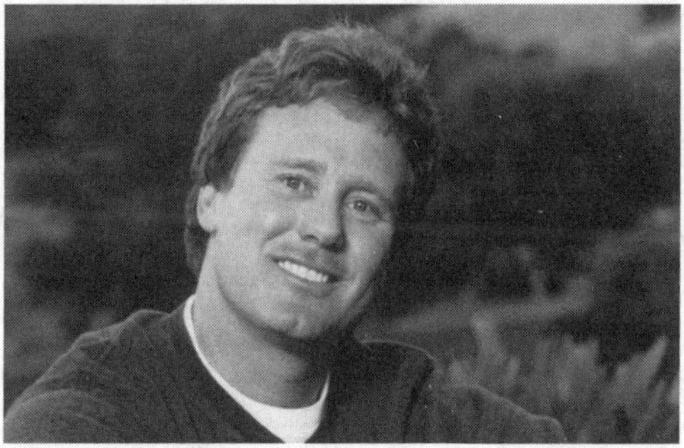

During his life, **Richard Carlson, PhD**, was considered one of the foremost experts in happiness and stress reduction in the United States and around the world and was a frequent featured guest on such shows as *Oprah*, *The Today Show*, *The View*, NNC, CNN, Fox, PBS, and over 2,000 other shows. *Don't Sweat the Small Stuff* continued to be a publishing phenomenon, with over twenty titles in the brand franchise, two of which were coauthored with his beloved wife, Kris. Richard died of a pulmonary embolism in December 2006, at the age of forty-five.

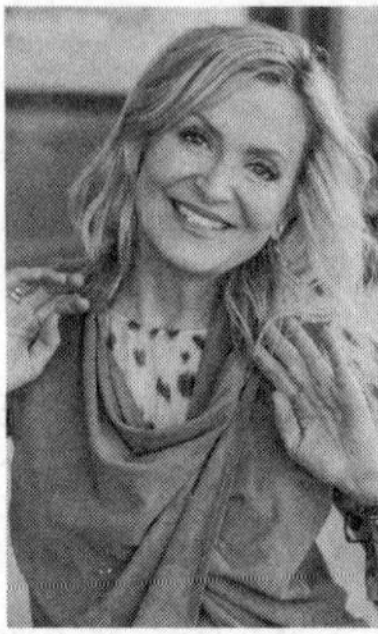

Alyssa Martens Photography

Kristine Carlson is a *New York Times* bestselling author and renowned speaker recognized worldwide for the global success of the Don't Sweat the Small Stuff book series she coauthored with her late husband, Dr. Richard Carlson. *Heartbroken Open*, Kristine's life-changing memoir, has become a biopic Lifetime Television movie starring Heather Locklear. The movie is titled *Don't Sweat the Small Stuff: The Kristine Carlson Story.*

With over twenty-five million books in print, Kristine has emerged today as a leading mindfulness expert and transformational guide who has been featured on national radio and television broadcasts, including *The Today Show*, *The View*, and *The Oprah Winfrey Show*. In 2010, she was awarded the Kennedy Laureate Award by John F. Kennedy University alongside the iconic chef Alice Waters and CNN's Dr. Sanjay Gupta.

In addition to her books *Don't Sweat the Small Stuff for Women*, *Don't Sweat the Small Stuff in Love*, and *Don't Sweat the Small Stuff for Moms*, Kristine's other titles include *An Hour to Live, An Hour to Love* and *From Heartbreak to Wholeness: The Hero's Journey to Joy*, her seminal self-help book for leading readers out of the pain of loss and into a new future.

Through her beloved women's retreats, including her signature What Now? program, Kristine serves as a guide for women navigating transition and change of all kinds—showing them how to live their most vibrant, joyous, and fulfilling life in their next chapter.

Through her popular podcast *Don't Sweat the Small Stuff, Live the Big Stuff,* Kristine's depth, realness, and ever-present humor shine through in each memorable episode. Her popular video-based Don't Sweat the Small Stuff Happiness Training Courses (on Dontsweat.com) teach people how to find inspiration and direction right in the midst of life's uncertainties—helping individuals around the world move from overwhelm and anxiety to an abiding optimism and trust in life. These courses feature exclusive video footage of Dr. Richard Carlson.

Kristine's mission is to show people that it is possible to love your life again after profound loss and major change—and to discover that more laughter, love, and happiness await you.